To my greatest father, my greatest mother, my brothers, and my sisters; to my husband, who gave all the best and supported me in all my decisions; to my best friends: Alryah, Awadya, and Nahla; and to my loving children.

Fathia Saeed Salih Mohamed

PROMOTION OF NURSING PRE AND POST OPEN HEART SURGERY

Post-Operative Care for Cardiothoracic Patients

AUSTIN MACAULEY PUBLISHERS™
LONDON * CAMBRIDGE * NEW YORK * SHARJAH

Copyright © Fathia Saeed Salih Mohamed 2022

The right of Fathia Saeed Salih Mohamed to be identified as author of this work has been asserted by the author in accordance with Federal Law No. (7) of UAE, Year 2002, Concerning Copyrights and Neighboring Rights.

All rights reserved. No part of this publication may be reproduced, stored in a retrieval system, or transmitted in any form or by any means, electronic, mechanical, photocopying, recording, or otherwise, without the prior permission of the publishers.

Any person who commits any unauthorized act in relation to this publication may be liable to legal prosecution and civil claims for damages.

The medical information in this book is not advice and should not be treated as such. Do not substitute this information for the medical advice of physicians. The information is general and intended to better inform readers of their health care. Always consult your doctor for your individual needs.

The age group that matches the content of the books has been classified according to the age classification system issued by the National Media Council.

ISBN – 9789948043706 – (Paperback)
ISBN – 9789948043713 – (Paperback)

Application Number: MC-10-01-0245374
Age Classification: E

Printer Name: iPrint Global Ltd
Printer Address: Witchford, England

First Published 2022
AUSTIN MACAULEY PUBLISHERS FZE
Sharjah Publishing City
P.O Box [519201]
Sharjah, UAE
www.austinmacauley.ae
+971 655 95 202

Table of Contents

Abstract	**19**
Chapter One: Introduction	**24**
1.1. History of Cardiac Surgery:	24
1.2. Justification	27
1.3. Objectives	27
1.3.1. General Objective	27
1.3.2. Specific Objectives	28
Chapter Two: Literature Review	**29**
2.1. Types of cardiac patients who should be treated surgically	29
2.2. Indications for valve replacement	30
2. Patients with ischemic heart disease	30
2.3. Surgical treatment for cardiac diseases	31
2.4. Post-operative assessment	32
2.4.1. Cardiovascular system	32
2.4.2. Respiratory system	33
2.4.3. Nervous	33
2.4.4. Renal	33

2.4.5. Gastrointestinal system	33
2.4.6. Pain	33
2.4.7. Wound	33
2.5. Postoperative management	34
2.5.1. Immediate nursing care for post-operative patient	34
2.5.2. Monitoring	35
2.5.3. Complication of cardiac surgery	38
2.5.3.1. Early post-operative period	38
2.5.3.2. Late postoperative period	38
2.5.3.2.1. Nursing intervention to prevent alter cardiac output	38
2.5.3.2.2. Nursing intervention to prevent impaired gas exchange	39
2.5.3.2.3. Nursing intervention to prevent bleeding	39
2.5.3.2.4. Nursing intervention for effective coping	39
2.5.4. Setting of intensive care unit for post-operative cardiac patient ICU	40
2.5.4.1. Components of ICU	40
2.5.4.2. Factors to consider	40
2.5.4.3. Location	40
2.5.4.4. Environment	41

2.5.4.5. Equipments	42
2.5.4.6. Personnel	42
2.5.5. Policy protocols and procedure	42
2.5.5.1. Policy	42
2.5.5.2. Procedure	42
2.5.5.3. Protocols	43
2.6. Infection Control	43
2.7. Documentation	43
2.8. Procedure used postoperative cardiac patients	44
2.8.1. End tracheal suction	44
2.8.2. Nursing intervention to facilitate suction	45
2.8.3. Patient assessment related to suction	45
2.8.3.1. Assessment Includes	45
2.8.4. End Tracheal Tube Management (ETT)	46
2.8.4.1. Equipments	46
2.8.4.2. Nursing Management	46
2.8.5. Chest Tube Management	47
2.8.5.1. Indications of Chest Tube Placement	47
2.8.5.2. Assessment for Caring of Patients with Chest Tube	47
How Are Chest Tubes Maintained?	48
2.8.5.3. Oxygen Administration Purpose	48

2.8.5.4. Equipments	48
2.8.5.5. Procedure	48
2.8.6. Central Venous Pressure (CVP) Indications	49
2.8.6.1. Preparations	49
2.8.6.2. Equipments	50
2.8.6.3. Procedures	50
2.8.6.4. CVP Measurements	50
2.8.7. Acid Base Balance and Arterial Blood Gases	51
2.8.7.1. Respiratory Acidosis	51
2.8.7.2. Metabolic Acidosis	52
2.8.7.3. Respiratory Alkalosis	52
2.8.7.2.4. Metabolic Alkalosis	52
2.8.8. Mechanical Ventilation	52
2.8.8.1. PEEP (Positive End – Expiratory Pressure)	53
2.8.8.2. Control Ventilation Mode	53
2.8.8.3. Assist Control Mode (A/C)	53
2.8.8.4. Synchronize Intermittent Mandatory Ventilation (SIMV)	53
2.9. Previous Studies	54
2.9.1. Training and education	58

Chapter Three: Methodology   **60**

   3.1. Study Design   60

     3.2. Study Area   60

     3.3. Study Population   61

     3.4. Inclusion Criteria   61

     3.5. Exclusion Criteria   61

     3.6. Sample Size   61

     3.7. Sampling Technique   61

     3.8. Methods of Data Collection   61

     3.9. Operational Definitions of Demographic Variables   62

     3.10. Study Instrument   64

   3.11. Phases of The Study   64

     3.11.1. Phase 1 (Monitoring and Supervision Procedure)   66

     3.11.2. Phase 2 (Training)   66

     3.11.3. Phase 3 (Evaluation)   67

     3.12. Ethical Considerations   68

     3.13. Data Analysis   68

Chapter Four: Discussion   **75**

Chapter Five: Conclusion and Recommendations   **82**

   6.1. Conclusion   82

     6.2. Recommendations   83

Reference	**84**
Appendices	**86**
Appendix (1)	86
Questionnaire	86
Appendix (2) Observation Checklist	117
Appendix (3) Education Program	132
Cont. Appendix (3.1) Continuing Professional Development Center	140

List of Table

Table (3.1): Operational Definitions of Variable	62
Table (4.1): Effect of Training on Nurses Performance Regarding Gastrointestinal Procedures.	69
Table (4.3): Effect of Training on Nurses' Performance Regarding Vascular Procedures.	70
Table (4.3): Effect of Training on Nurses' Performance Regarding Vascular Procedures.	71
Table (4.4): Effect of Training on Nurses' Performance Regarding Dressing Procedure.	72
Table (4.5): Effect of Training on Nurses' Performance Regarding Activities of Living.	74

List of Appendices

Questionnaire	86
Observation Checklist	117
Education Program	132
Continuing Professional Development Center	140

الملاحق العربية

ملحق (1.1): طريقة قياس الضغط الوريدي المركزي		89
ملحق (3.1): العناية بالمريض على جهاز التنفس الصناعي		97
ملحق (4.1): كيفية العناية بالجرح الناتج من إجراء عملية جراحية		100
ملحق (5.1): طريقة قياس الضغط الوريدي المركزي		104
ملحق (6.1): العناية بمريض متصل بقسطرة وريد مركزية		106
ملحق (7.1): العناية بمريض متصل بكانيولا شريانية		109
ملحق (8.1): طريقة قياس ضغط الدم الشرياني المباشر بواسطة جهاز المونيتور		112
ملحق (9.1): العناية بمريض متصل بأنبوبة صدرية		114
ملحق (1.2): قائمة مراجعة لتقييم أداء الممرضات في العلامات الحيوية		123
ملحق (2.2): التنفس وقياس ضغط الدم		126
ملحق (3.2): قائمة مراجعة لتقييم أداء الممرضات في الإنقاذ عن طريق إنعاش القلب (فردين)		129

From the bottom of my heart, I convey my sincere thanks to my main supervisor: Prof. Magda Elhadi Ahmed Yousif and to my co-supervisor, Mr. Ahmed Sayed Ahmed, the head manager of Alshaab teaching hospital, who supported and connected me with the continuous professional development center for training program.

I acknowledge with great appreciation the valuable help given to me by the nursing staff, in Ahmed Gasim and Alshaab teaching hospital.

List of Abbreviation

A&E	Accident and emergency
AMI	Acute myocardial infarction
ASD	A trial septal defect
CCRN	Critical care registered nurse
CCU	Coronary care unit
CO	Cardiac out put
CO	HR X S.V
CPAP	Continuous positive airway pressure
CVA	Cerebrovascular accident
CVD	Cerebrovascular diseases
ECG	Electrocardiogram
EMS	Emergency medical services
HR	Heart rate
IABP	Intraortic balloon pumps
ICCU	Intensive cardiac care unit
IV	Intraviend
LDL	Low-density lipoprotein
MI	Myocardial infarction
NCP	Nursing care plan
P.D.A	Patent duteous arterious
PCI	Percutaneous coronary intervention
PEEP	Positive end expiratory pressure
PT	Bleeding time

PTT	Platelet count
S.V.	Stroke volume
SIMV	Synchronize intermittent mandatory ventilation
SPSS	Statistical package for social sciences
STEMI	St.segment elevation myocardial
SVO2	Venous ox hemoglobin saturationnitor
UA	Unstable angina
USA	Untied estate of American
V.S.D	Ventricular septal defect
WHO	World health organization

Abstract

Open heart surgery is a critical surgery so the team should be qualified enough to deal with the patient who needs intensive care, the care that is provided to a patient who requires close observation or specialized treatments that cannot be provided in general ward. This pre- and post-interventional study conducted in Alshaab and Ahmed Gasim cardiac center. The aim of this study was to promote nursing management post open heart surgery. The study population was 98 nurses representing a total coverage of all nurses who work in intensive cardiac care unit not less than six months. They were used over six months. The data collected through interview and observation check list were used over six months, the variables were the procedures which should be done for the patient after open heart surgery. A special designed questionnaire was filled and an observation check list with steps of every procedure was done according to US National Database of nursing quality indicators (guidelines for data collection – the American Nurses Association). The intervention was conducted in continuing professional development and training center in Khartoum in addition to the practical training in cardiac centers. To compare and describe the results descriptive analysis was performed using Chi-square test. The results show that the level of knowledge (urgent care post-operative (pre86% poor, post 84% excellent). Arterial blood gases knowledge (31% poor pre, 86% excellent post), dealing with endotracheal tube (52% poor pre, post 82% excellent). Role of nursing with chest tube (59% poor pre, 86% post excellent). Chest tube removal (40% poor pre, 95%excellent post). Care with ventilator device (pre 43% poor, 85% excellent post). The findings here are realistic and indicate the way into which nurses comply with the training-protocol, however there is inadequate monitoring and closed supervision of nursing practice. In these observations the investigator concluded that training as an intervention was the most influential factor in nurses performance as they will be able to provide an excellent service if they are trained. Supervised, and have incentives to practice properly. The study recommended the increase of the number of nurses to the rate of one nurse to one patient and setting a protocol to improve knowledge and critical care nursing courses.

الخلاصة

إنَّ جراحة القلب هي جراحة خطيرة؛ لذا يجب أن يكون الفريق مؤهلاً بصورة كافية ليتعامل مع المرضى الذين يحتاجون عناية مركَّزة، وهي العناية التي تُقدَّم للمريض الذي يتطلَّب مراقبة لصيقة أو معالجات متخصصة، والتي لا تقدم في العنبَر العام. أجريت هذه الدراسة ذات التدخل القَبْلِيّ والبَعدِيّ في مركزَي: أحمد قاسم والشعب للقلب. كان هدف الدراسة هو ترقية الرعاية التمريضية عقب جراحة القلب. عدد مجتمع الدراسة كان 98 ممرضة، تمَّت التغطية الكاملة لكل الممرضات اللائي يعملن بوحدات العناية القلبية المركزية، لفترة لا تقل عن ستة أشهر. تم اختيارهن وفقاً لطريقة التغطية الشاملة. ولجمع البيانات تمَّ استخدام المقابلة، وقائمة تحديد الملاحظات لِمدَّة ستَّةِ أشهر، وكانَت المتغيِّرات هي الإجراءات التي يجب أنْ تُعمَل للمريض عقب

جراحة القلب المفتوح. تم ملء استبيان معهم بطريقة خاصة، وعمل قائِمة تحديدِ الملاحظة مَعَ خطوات الإجراءات اللازمة وفقاً لقاعدة البيانات الأمريكية القومية لمؤشرات جودة التمريض (الخطوط التوجيهية لجمع البيانات – جمعية الممرضات الأميركية). أُجرِي التدخُّل في مركز التطوير المهني المستمر بالخرطوم، إضافة إلى التدريب العملي في مراكز القلب. وبوصف ومقارنة النتائج، تم أداء التحليل الوصفي بواسطة اختيار مربع كأي. أظهرت النتائج أن المستوى المعرفي (للرعاية العاجلة عقب العملية. 86% ضعيف قبل، 84% ممتاز بعد) معرفة غازات الدم الشرياني (31 ضعيف قبل، 86% ممتاز بعد)، فيما يتعلق بالأنبوب داخل الرغامَى (52% ضعيف قبل، 82% ممتاز بعد) رعاية جهاز التنفس (43% ضعيف قبل، 85% ممتاز بعد) المخرجات هنا حقيقية وتشير إلى الطريقة التي يمتثل بها الممرضات مع نظام التدريب، ولكن الرقابة والمراقبة اللصيقة لممارسة التمريض غير كافية، هذه الملاحظات، خلصت الباحثة إلى أن التدريب كتدخُّل، كان العامل الأكثر تأثيراً في أداء الممرضات، حيث إنهن كن قادرات على توفير خدمة ممتازة إذا تم تدريبهن

والإشراف عليهنَّ، وكان لديهن حوافز للممارسة الصحيحة. أوصَتِ الدراسة بزيادة عدد الممرضات بنسبة ممرض لكل مريض، وبوضع بروتوكول لتحسين المعرفة ودورات تدريبية للتمريض في الحالات الحرجة.

Chapter One
Introduction

Cardiovascular surgery is a surgery on the heart and/or great vessels performed by cardiac surgeons. Frequently, it is done to treat complications of ischemic heart disease, it also includes heart transplantation.

The specialty of cardiovascular surgical nursing has developed advanced and improved care of patients before and after the operation and is now well established. The experiences of the cardiovascular surgical are to the ultimate recovery of the patient, and prevent complications.

1.1 History of Cardiac Surgery:

On July 10, 1893, Dr. Daniel Hale Williams, a surgeon from Chicago, successfully operated on a 24-year-old man who had been stabbed in the heart during a fight. The patient was admitted to Chicago's provident hospital on July 9 at 7:30 P.M., the stab wound was slightly on left of the sternum and dead center over the heart. Initially, the wound was thought to be superficial, but during the night, the patient experience persistent bleeding, pain, and profound symptoms of shock. Williams opened the patient's chest and tied off an artery and vein that had been injured inside the chest wall, likely causing the blood loss. Then he noticed a tear in the pericardium and a puncture wound to the heart, "about one-tenth of an inch in length." American heart association guidelines for cardiopulmonary http://circ.ahajournals-89.

The wound in the right ventricle was not bleeding, so Williams did not place a stitch through the heart wound. He did, however, stitch closed the hole in the pericardium. The patient recovered. Williams reported this case 4 years later. This operation, which is referred to frequently, is probably the first successful surgery involving a documented stab wound to heart. At the time, Williams surgery was considered bold and daring, and although he did not actually place a stitch through the wound in the heart, his treatment seems to have been appropriate. Under the circumstances, he most likely saved the patient's life.

A few years after Williams case, a couple of other surgeons actually sutured heart Germany, performed what many consider the first successful heart operation. On September 7, 1896, a 22-year-old man was stabbed in the heart and collapsed. The police found him pale, covered with cold sweat, and extremely short of breath. His pulse was irregular, and his clothes were soaked with blood. By September 9, his condition was worsening, as shown in Dr. Rehn's case note.

The cardiac surgery patient is critical who needs close observation so special staff of nursing should be available and special area advance supplies for monitoring and saving file.

The recognition and subsequent of intensive care began in 1950, and was influenced by a number of factors, significantly the development of cardiac surgery with requirement for post-operative care (American heart association).

Over the last three decades, the specialty of critical care and profession of nursing has interacted in some very important ways. Clearly, care as a nursing specialty has had an important impact on the profession. When critical care evolved in the late 1960, nurses working in intensive care unit developed knowledge level and confidence rarely seen in the hospital setting.

The focus of critical care nursing is to provide care for the patients who are experiencing a life-threatening or potentially life-threatening illness or injury (American heart association, 2006).

The nursing care that provided is intended to restore health, alleviate suffering, pain, and preserve the rights and dignity of individuals.

The care of critically ill patient is becoming increasingly more complex, and critical care nurses need a quick reference to consult for answer to many questions about patient disease process. Key assessment criteria, therapies and patient care issues (Lee, 2006).

In caring post-operative cardiac critically ill patient, nurses continuously observe and monitor the patient for physiological alteration. They also plan to carry out intervention that compensate for altered body functioning and recognize both complications and important response to therapeutic modalities.

With advancement in biomedical technology, diagnostic and clinical therapeutics, critically ill patients are treated in complex and highly charged milieu.

Cardiac surgery requires critical care nurses who have a broad knowledge base, demonstrate expert clinical and decision-making skill, and share commitment to nursing ethical and professional values.

The practice base for critical care nursing requires knowledge from the biological, behavioral, social, and nursing domains (Caral, 2001).

1.2 Justification

To the best of knowledge of the researcher, there are no research studies about promotion of nursing regarding open-heart surgery therefore, it is necessary to conduct this study to assess the effect of trained nurses in critical cardiac unit post open-heart surgery.

According to the result from a previous study that stated high mortality rates among cardiac surgery patients, and deficiency in critical care nursing in Sudan in ministry of health report (2009). A study was conducted between 2009 and 2013 to promote nurses knowledge and practice in intensive cardiac care unit.

1.3 Objectives

1.3.1 General Objective

To promote nurses knowledge, practices, and attitudes regarding nursing care post- operative cardiac patients in ICU in Al Shaab and Ahmed Gasim Cardiac Centers.

1.3.2 Specific Objectives

- To assess nurses knowledge, practice, and attitude about critical care for post- operative cardiac patients.
- To promote nurses skills to prevent complications that may occur.
- To assess the training effect on nurses performance to be expert.
- To change behavior and attitude.

Chapter Two
Literature Review

Critical care nursing is the care provided to patients of all ages with alterations in physical and emotional health. Intensive care is the care provided to a patient who requires close observation or specialized treatments that cannot be provided in the general ward.

2.1 Types of cardiac patients who should be treated surgically

1. Patients with a symptomatic valve disease: valve replacement

The disease affecting the cardiac valves often leads to severe functional limitations for patient due to either a stenotic or regurgitate change in the valve function.

Most commonly, the mitral and aortic valves are involved because of higher pressure generates by the left side of the heart.

2.2 Indications for valve replacement

- Mitral stenosis

Usually the result of rheumatic fever but also be caused by tumor.

- Mitral regurgitation

Result of rheumatic disease, mitral valve prolapsed and endocarditis (Caral, 2001). Surgery indicated in symptomatic patients when a pressure gradient 0.50 MHG or more is present across the cardiac aortic valve.

Aortic stenosis caused by rheumatic inflammation, idiopathic calcification and congenital malformation.

- Aortic regurgitation

The most common cause is endocarditis and blunt chest trauma.

There are tissue valves or mechanical replacement.

2. Patients with ischemic heart disease

- Coronary artery by passes graft – CABG

The rationale of CABG is to restore adequate blood flow and to provide nutritional support to myocardial tissue.

- Indication of CABG

- Chronic stable angina refractory to medical therapy.
- Significant left main coronary occlusion 75 percent.
- Triple vessel coronary artery disease.

- Unstable angina pectoris.
- Acute myocardial infarction.
- Emergent.
- Delayed.
- Left ventricular failure.
- Congestive heart failure.
- Carcinogenic shock (Cabello et al., 2010).

3. Patients with vascular emergency:

Abdominal aoric aneurysm, acute arterial occlusion are indicated for surgery as vascular emergency.

Congenital heart diseases are cause for cardiac surgery.

Ventricular sepal defect (V.S.D) a trial sepal defect patent ductus (P.D.A) altlreroses and tetrology of float are common.

4. Patients with congenital heart disease indicated for surgery:

Ventricular sepal defect V.S.D
Arterial septal defect
Patent duct altlreroses (P.D.A)
Tetrology of flout.

2.3 Surgical treatment for cardiac diseases

Surgical treatment for cardiac disease continues to provide a significant challenge to nurses in the management of these patients.

All medical staff collaborates on the management of the cardiac throughout the post-operative recovery phase.

During the acute post-operative phase patient are monitored continuously as systemic recovery from anesthesia occurs and body temperature return to normal (Caral, 2001).

The primary goals of nursing management are to ensure the adequacy of the cardiac index, tissue perfusion, and monitor neurologic recovery.

Systemic responses to the operative procedure and the cardiopulmonary pump run are monitored.

Nursing management of the patient is accomplished through monitoring of the direct and derived hemodynamic parameters, clinical assessment, and laboratory.

The focus of nursing management of the patients continues assessment and prompt intervention to maintain on adequate cardiac index to meet metabolic need.

Concurrently the critical nurse assists the family in coping with the situation crisis of the illness, receiving communications about the patient's progress, and verbalizing their feeling (Canto et al., 2007).

2.4 Post-operative assessment

2.4.1 Cardiovascular system

Cardiac rate and rhythm oxygen saturation peripheral blood pressure central venous pressure PAP/LAP cardiac output temperature fluid coagulation status, ECG rate, and rhythm, edema, synopsis, and urine output.

2.4.2 Respiratory system

Patient should be assessed for air entry, breath sound, secretions placement of endotracheal tube, setting on ventilator arterial blood gases chest tube system.

Also patients should be assessed for restlessness, cyanosis, rapid rate unequal chest expansion for ineffective ventilation.

2.4.3 Nervous

Pupil size, reaction orientation, and level of consciousness motor functioning.

2.4.4 Renal

Urinary output urine, character, color, specific gravity electrolytes.

2.4.5 Gastrointestinal system

Nasogastric secretions bowel sound (Canto, 2007)

2.4.6 Pain

Quality, intensity location integumentary skin breakdown incisional healing and drainage.

2.4.7 Wound

Assessing wound for bleeding and infection.

2.5 Postoperative management

The goal of post-operative care is to:

- Maintain good level of oxygenation and carbon dioxide.
- Hemodynamic stability and adequate organ perfusion.
- Prevent and reduce atalactasis.
- Prevent cerebral dysfunction.
- Prevent adequate analgesis.
- Maintain fluid and electrolyte balance.
- Appropriate and problem-free extubation (Caral, 2001).

2.5.1 Immediate nursing care for post-operative patient

Irrespective of the cardiac function all patients returning to the intensive care unit after an open-heart surgery are in a state of controlled shock due to fluid shift and varying vascular tone.

The primary goals of management are to ensure the adequacy of the cardiac index and leisure perfusion and monitor neurological recovery. Systemic responses are monitored.

Immediately after arrival to I.C.U, 100% oxygen is given through the end tracheal tube supported with the mechanical ventilator.

- Patient assessment for ABC (airway, breathing, circulation).

- Pliers connected to monitor for arterial pressure monitoring.
- E.C.G., arterial blood pressure (ABP), arterial and central venues pressure (C.V.P) measurement.
- Assessment of cardiothoracic tube for bleeding.
- Fluid administration is maintained, and intake & output.
- Blood sample are taken for arterial blood gas and serum electrolytes.
- Portable chest radiography is taken.
- Monitoring cardiac output (co), which is represented by the following formulae:-
  CO=HR X S.V
  CO=cardiac out put
  HR=Heart Rate
  SV=Stroke VOLUME (Caral, 2001).

2.5.2 Monitoring

The nurse collects the baseline data on cardiovascular status by checking the following parameters:

1. **Heart rate and rhythm**: continuous ECG monitoring is carried out.

2. **Peripheral pulses**: assessment of peripheral pulses in all extremities is important, is focused in maintaining a sinus rhythm. In certain patients it may be necessary to use trial-pacing wires to get rid of the dys-arrhythmias.

3. **Arterial blood pressure**: for all critically ill patients a minimum mean arterial pressure 50-55 mm of Hg is maintained to adequate overall systemic perfusion and cerebral and renal perfusion. Normally arterial blood pressure is continuously monitored in the peripheral vessel such as redial artery.

4. **Cardiac filling pressure**: cardiac filling pressure assesses the cardiac performance. It left a trial pressure catheter which provides a continuous approximation of left ventricular and diastolic pressure. The upper limit is 22-24 mm of Hg caution hound be taken to reach this level as it demands administration of fluid (Siley, 2001).

5. **Cardiac output**: a pulmonary artery catheter allows cardiac output measurement by thermo dilution technique. Cardiac output reading are converted to a cardiac index (CO divided by the body surface area). A cardiac index of 2.0 liters/min./m^2 or greater is sufficient to sufficient to maintain organ perfusion.

6. **Mixed venous ox hemoglobin saturation**: catheters are used to measure and display venous ox hemoglobin saturation (SVO2) in the pulmonary artery. Continuous display of SVO2 allows observation of change in cardiac performances. Equipment used for this should calibrate.

7. **Ventilatory parameters**: are monitored during the post-operative period. If the ventilator function is adequate and the patient has adequate spontaneous breathing, patient is weaned from ventilator within 24 hours.

8. **Arterial blood gases, acid base status**: regular of arterial blood gas and acid base is done during the postoperative to period to ensure the ventilator function and acid base status.

9. **Serum electrolytes**: measurement of potassium and calcium help to prevent problems especially when the value is lower borderline. K replacements are mandatory if serum K is low. Infusion of calcium chloride improves cardiac function. During post-operative period maintenance of serum potassium is vital. Serum potassium value should be measured frequently to guide replacement therapy.

10. **Urine output**: in the initial post-operative period urine output is increased whereas it diminishes between 8-12 the post CPB hours. Urine output should be maintained approximately 1 ml/kg/hour. Maintaining of this level is achieved by using furosemide or mannitol. Cardiac filling pressure guides diuretic therapy (Siley, 2001)

2.5.3 Complication of cardiac surgery
2.5.3.1 Early post-operative period

Acute MI, cardiac dys-arrhythmias, hemorrhage, pulmonary embolism fever, depression electrolyte, disturbances systemic arterial hypertension, cerebral infarcts, confusion, disseminated intravascular coagulation, acute respiratory distress syndrome, and renal failure.

2.5.3.2 Late postoperative period

Wound infection, post pericardiotomy syndrome. Systemic arterial emboli, infective endocarditic and occlusion of graft (Jaya, 2008).

2.5.3.2.1 Nursing intervention to prevent alter cardiac output

Monitor cardiac direct and indirect parameters, dys-arrhythmias, and oxygen saturation, SVO2. Blood pressure urine output, level of sensorium tissue perfusion monitor peripheral pulses and capillary refill anticipate volume replacement using colloid/ crystalloid/ blood and products.

Return slowly monitoring temperature observe for shivering restlessness, initiate temporary pacing if indicated monitor arterial blood gas, K+, mg and vital signs.

Administer antiarrhythmic drugs as ordered.

Monitor cardiac enzymes and ECG.

Monitor chest tube drainage and report abnormal findings such as change in drainage, widening mediastinum and change in BP.

2.5.3.2.2 Nursing intervention to prevent impaired gas exchange

Monitor ABG values and ventilator settings in the presence of secretions, suction using oxygenation, hyperinflation, suction, and inflation techniques.

Monitor SaO2, FLO2, peep levels. Monitor muscle strength respiratory effort, hemodynamic parameters, heart rate and anxiety levels.

Monitor clinical readiness for weaning turn the patient every 2 hours monitor hydration status encourage progressive activity ambulation as condition allows provide analgesia (Jaya, 2008).

2.5.3.2.3 Nursing intervention to prevent bleeding

- Monitor PT, PTT, bleeding time platelet count.
- Anticipate and prepare for transfusion.
- Monitor chest tube drainage and report increase in drainage more than 100ml/2hour maintain chest tube patency.
- Assess drainage system.

2.5.3.2.4 Nursing intervention for effective coping

Introduce oneself to family members, conduct family assessment, ensure that family's needs are met, ensure clear communication, encourage the family verbalizing this fear and anxiety, evaluate the ability to cope, support the patient throughout period of anxiety period adequate explanations (Suzan, 1995).

2.5.4 Setting of intensive care unit for post-operative cardiac patient ICU

- The critical ill patent is the patient who is experiencing a life-threatening or potentially life-threatening illness or injury.

- The patient who admitted to cardiac ICU are all post-operative cardiac patients they are not weaning from mechanical ventilator.

- The objective of intensive care unit setting is to provide functional and user-friendly environment.

2.5.4.1 Components of ICU

- Consistent monitoring.
- Rapid skill intervention, and
- Multidisciplinary team work.

2.5.4.2 Factors to consider

- Sources of patient.
- Admission and discharge criteria.
- Expected rate of occupancy.
- Personal required.
- Technological resources.

2.5.4.3 Location

- The location should be chosen so that the unit is adjacent to direct elevator enabling travelling to and

from emergency department, operating room, intermediate care unit, and the radiology department.
- Patients must be situated so that direct or indirect visualization of health care providers is possible at all time (Suzan, 1995).
- Bed strength
- Ideally 8 to 12 beds.
- One isolated bed for every ten beds.
- Bed space is 150 to 200 square feet per bed.

2.5.4.4 Environment

- Floor coverings and ceiling with sound absorption properties.
- Doorway offset to minimize sound transmission.
- Light and soft music except 10 P.M. to 6 A. M.
- Air conditioning, split and central.
- Cleaning: vacuum cleaning and wet mopping of floor.
- Windows are import aspect of sensory orientation also clock and calendar and pillow speaker connected to radio and television are improving orientation.
- Electrical, water, and gas must be adequate.
- Hand washing area and disposable paper towels.
- Telephone and computer for communication.
- Sterilizing area, waste, and sharp disposable.

There should be a separate medication area of at least 50 square feet containing a refrigerator, also a table for preparation of drugs (Bartom, 2005).

2.5.4.5 Equipments

- Monitoring equipment.
- Therapeutic equipment.
- Audio and visual alarm, battery backup and charging.

2.5.4.6 Personnel

- Nurse ratio 1 to 1.
- ICU manager.
- A registered nurse with BCN or preferably and MNS degree, certification in critical care or equivalent graduate education with at least 2 years' experience working in critical care unit.
- Medical staffing cover for every shift (Bartom, 2005).

2.5.5 Policy protocols and procedure
2.5.5.1 Policy

Policy is a course of action for dealing a particular matter or a situation by political party, government or an organization.

2.5.5.2 Procedure

Procedure is a set of action necessary for doing something.

2.5.5.3 Protocols

It is the ceremonial system of fixed roles and accepted behaviors especially used by companies, institutions, and organization.

The critical care to maintain uniformity and ensure quality (Bartom, 2005).

There should be clear-cut policies regarding admission and discharge, transfer, emergency, safety procedures, and infection control.

2.6 Infection Control

- Surveillance.
- Sterilization.
- Quality control and auditing.

2.7 Documentation

- Conventional.
- Electronic medical record.
- Bedside terminals interfaced with existing hospital data system and data retrieval like laboratory result and x-ray report.
- Remote data transmission capabilities – to office and on call room.

2.8 Procedure used postoperative cardiac patients

2.8.1 End tracheal suction

Suctioning is the mechanical aspiration of oral and pulmonary secretions for the purpose of maintaining patent airway. It is a sterile procedure.

- Indication

It is indicated whenever a patient is unable to clear secretion.

Independently preparation for extubation, assessment of airway patency, coughs reflex stimulation, and sputum specimen collection.

- Technique recommended for section

The section catheter is placed through an artificial airway into the tracheal and intermittent negative pressure is applied only as the catheter is withdrawn.

- To prevent aspiration of mucosa withdrawn the catheter approximately one cent before applying the section.
- Rotate the catheter in smooth, constant motion. Each pass should be no more than 10 second.
- Limit suction passes to the minimal number.
- Minimal recover time between suction passes should be (20-30) seconds.

2.8.2 Nursing intervention to facilitate suction

- Position the patient to facilitate coughing.
- Assess the patient and treated before suction.
- Encourage the patient to take deep breath before coughing.
- Assess tube patency.
- Maintaining a septic technique.

2.8.3 Patient assessment related to suction

The patient should be assessed before, during and after suctioning.

2.8.3.1 Assessment Includes

- Respiration (rate, depth, change).
- Work of breathing.
- Breath sound.
- Cough character and ability to expectorate.
- Sputum amount, color and odder.
- Oxygen saturation.
- Vital sign.
- Intracranial pressure.
- Arterial blood gas-skin for color and temperature.

2.8.4 End Tracheal Tube Management (ETT)
2.8.4.1 Equipments

- Endotracheal tube.
- Stylet.
- Laryngoscope with functioning light.
- A syringe for checking and inflating the pilot for the cuff.
- A tape for securing the endotracheal tube after placement (Bartom, 2005).

2.8.4.2 Nursing Management

- Monitoring and record the ETT size and c m mark where the tube exist the patient tip, teeth, or nostril which help to detect accidental advancement or dislodgement or dislodgement of the ETT.
- Assessment for and prevention of the skin breakdown related to ETT pressure.
- Maintaining a patent ETT by suctioning as needed and providing warm and humidified gases.
- Providing comfort measure and minimizing anxiety with analgesia, sedation repositioning, and ongoing communication with the patient.

2.8.5 Chest Tube Management
2.8.5.1 Indications of Chest Tube Placement

- Post thoracic surgery (after open-heart surgery chest tubes are place in the mediastinum toc remove residual blood or drainage)
- Pneumothorax
- Hemothorax.
- Bronchopleural fistula
- Penetrating chest injury
- Empyema (Jaya, 2008).

2.8.5.2 Assessment for Caring of Patients with Chest Tube

- Assessment of chest tube should be done at least once a shift and with any sudden change.
- Assessment of hemodynamic and respiratory status.
- The amount color, consistency of the chest drainage should be assessed and documented.
- The chest tube insertion site should be assessed during every shift or as clinically indicated.
- Monitor the water seal chamber for pulping (continuous pulping indicates leak in the system).
- Assessing the system for the sources of an air leak.

How Are Chest Tubes Maintained?

- Chest tube connections should be taped and secured
- The drainage unit should be below the level of the chest tube insertion site ideally 2-3 feet below chest level
- Chest tube dressing should be clean, dry and occlusive and mote any drainage on dressing and reinforce as needed
- Change the drainage requires clamped (Jaya, 2008).

2.8.5.3 Oxygen Administration Purpose

- To supply oxygen in conditions when there is an interference with normal oxygenation of blood.
- To reduce the effect of anoxaemia.
- To maintain health level in tissue oxygenation.

2.8.5.4 Equipments

- Oxygen supply with flow meter.
- Humidifier with sterile distilled water.
- Oxygen mask or nasal cannula.
- Tape if needed to secure the cannula in place.
- Gauze to pad the tubing over the neck.

2.8.5.5 Procedure

- Determine the need for oxygen therapy.
- Assist the patient to semi-flower position as possible.

- Explain the procedure to the patient.
- Set up the oxygen equipment and humidified.
- Turn on the oxygen at the prescribed rate and ensure proper functioning.
- Slip gauze pads under the tubing over the neck bones to prevent skin irritation.
- Assess the patient regularly.
- Assess the vital sign, color, breathing patter and chest movement.
- Chest that the equipment are working regularly.
- Record initiation of therapy and all nursing assessments.

2.8.6 Central Venous Pressure (CVP)
Indications

- Central venous pressure reflects right ventricular failure.
- CVP is useful indication of adequacy of venous blood volume and alteration of cardiovascular function.
- Management of the patient on shock.

2.8.6.1 Preparations

- Explain the procedure to the patient.
- CVP site should be prepared by shaving and cleaning with an antiseptic solution.
- Measure the length of the manometer.
- Measure the length of the catheter required from anatomical puncture point to superior vena cava.

- Assemble articles required for the procedure.
- Place the patient in a comfortable position (Jaya, 2008).

2.8.6.2 Equipments

- Venous pressure apparatus with water manometer.
- Infusion solution and infusion catheter.
- Three-way stop clock.
- IV pole attached to bed arm board and adhesive tape.

2.8.6.3 Procedures

- Attach the manometer to the IV pole with the zero point of the monometer on the level with the patient right.
- Mark the mid axillary line on the patient which is the reference point for subsequent reading.
- The intravenous catheter is passed through median basilica, subclavian or jugular vein CVP catheter is connected to a three-way stopcock which communicates with the manometer and open IV system.
- Catheter is secured by suture to prevent accidental removal and apply dressing

2.8.6.4 CVP Measurements

- Always adjust the position of the patient to the position used for first reading.

- Position the zero point on the manometer with the level 0 of the atrium.
- Turn the stop clock so that the IV solution flows into the manometer filling 20-25 cm level.
- Turn the stop clock again so that the solution in the manometer flows into the patient (Jaya, 2008).
- Observe the fall of height of the fluid in the manometer, record the level at which it stabilizes.
- Turn the stop clock against to allow the IV solution to flow from the container to the patient vein by slow drip.
-

2.8.7 Acid Base Balance and Arterial Blood Gases

- Normal range of the blood is (7.35-7.45).
- Normal range of HCO_3 is (22-26).
- Normal range of CO_2 is (35-45).
- Acidosis occurs when the PH of the blood is below the normal range.
- Acidosis is classified as respiratory or metabolic, depending on what type of acid (CO_2 OR HCO_3) is present in an excess.

2.8.7.1 Respiratory Acidosis

Occurs with any process that decreases the rate of CO_2 gas exchange in alveolar ventilation.

2.8.7.2 Metabolic Acidosis

Is decrease in plasma bicarbonate concentration and PH related to an accumulation of acid or loss? (PH less than 7.35 and HCO3 less than 22).

Alkalosis occurs when PH is above normal (PH more than 45).

2.8.7.3 Respiratory Alkalosis

Is the result of hyperventilation and hypocpnia. PH more than 7.45 and PC2 less than 35.

2.8.7.2.4 Metabolic Alkalosis

Is excessive gain of base (from bicarbonate or anions metabolized to form bicarbonate) or loss of hydrogen ions.

PH more than 7.45 more than 26.

2.8.8 Mechanical Ventilation

With volume ventilation the desired tidal volume is delivered, regardless of the pressure required to do so, airway pressure reflects the pressure required to move gases down the airways (resistant) and to distend the lung and chest wall (compliance).

Pressure ventilation ensure a pre-selected pressure with each breath, volume varies with resistant and compliance.

2.8.8.1 PEEP (Positive End –Expiratory Pressure)

Peep is the team used when the patient receives positive pressure breath, used in patient with restrictive (noncompliance) disease, whereas CPAP (continues positive airway pressure) is a team used when the patient is breathing entirely on his or her own. CPAP is used to restore FRC during spontaneous breathing trials, and with patient with sleep apnea to provide pneumatic splint during sleep so that apneic episode secondary to airway occlusion prevented.

2.8.8.2 Control Ventilation Mode

It is needed only when the patient is unable to initiate spontaneous inspiration (e.g. sedated and paralyzed).

2.8.8.3 Assist Control Mode (A/C)

The clinician selects a control rate, aspiratory time, volume, sensitivity, FLO2, and PEEP if (desired). When the patient initiates breath between control breath, the ventilator delivers a full tidal volume.

2.8.8.4 Synchronize Intermittent Mandatory Ventilation (SIMV)

Tidal volume, mandatory rate, aspiratory time, sensitivity and FLO2 are set. PEEP is selected if desired. When the patient initiates a breath, the ventilator senses the effort and delivers air flow to the patient. The patient can breathe at his or her own rate and volume between the mandatory trial volumes breaths.

Synchronized refer to the ventilators attempts to deliver the mandatory breath within a certain period in synchrony with patient spontaneous breaths (Jaya, 2008).

2.9 Previous Studies

Coronary heart disease, the main cause of death today, the single largest killer worldwide. It has become a true pandemic and its incidence is still rising. According to the WHO, in 2002, 7.2 million deaths worldwide resulted from coronary heart disease. In many developed countries, especially in North America and Western European countries, coronary heart disease and resulting death rates are decreasing. This decrease is the result of improved prevention. Diagnosis and treatment, particularly reductions in cigarette smoking. Blood cholesterol and blood pressure, bellarmine college, (Caral, 2001).

Our purpose was to identify general information and nursing behaviors perceived as indicators of caring of patients who have had cardiac problem need surgical intervention. A sample of 22 hospitalized patients were interviewed, with use of an open-ended question and the caring behaviors assessment, to determine what things nurse said or did that convey caring to patients during their stay in the coronary care unit (CCU). An analysis of the relative importance of each identified behavior revealed that nursing actions that focused on the physical care and monitoring of patients were seen as most indicative caring. Teaching activities were also perceived as significant whereas extra, individualized aspects of care were viewed as important in the critical care setting. No significant differences in perceptions were found on the basis of sex, age, education level, number of CCU admissions, or length of CCU stay. Critical care nurses should be aware a general information's about disease and assessment activities and demonstration of care are viewed by patients as significant expressions of caring.

A randomized controlled trial of in-hospital nursing support for myocardial infarction patients and their partners: effects on anxiety and depression. D.R Thompson. Department of Nursing, University of Liverpool.

This study monitored and compared levels of anxiety and depression reported by myocardial infarction (MI) patients and their partners, throughout the patients' hospital stay. An independent variable of a programme of supportive-educative counseling provided by a coronary care nurse was introduced to determine whether it significantly affected reactions. Sixty couples were randomly assigned to one of two groups: (a) the treatment group, in which they received the systematic programme of nursing support in addition to routine care, or (b) the control group, in which they received routine care but no other intervention. Anxiety and depression were measured by the hospital anxiety and depression (HAD) scale at 24 hours and 5 days after the patient's admission to hospital. At 5 days there were statistically significant differences between both groups with respect to the HAD scale mean scores. These findings strongly suggest that a simple programme of in-hospital couple counseling, provided by a coronary care nurse, and statistically significantly reduce anxiety and depression in MI patients and anxiety in their partners.

Study of nursing care of cardiac patients in C.C.U. and A&E and the role of education and effective training in the optimization of the quality of healthcare in both department

Seyed Habibollah Kavari health management (Ph.D.), principal lecture of the medical school, Shiraz University, Shiraz, Iran (2003).

The results of this study are:

1. This evaluation of an interventional program detected improvement on the behavior, knowledge, and attitudes of CCU nurses.
2. After education program nurses are aware of how to practice suitable nursing care plan to care by coronary heart disease patients suffering from main symptoms chest pain, dyspnea, and potential complications.
3. A co-ordinate disease management approach may be implemented that includes assessment in the hospital, comprehensive education, and behavior modification in order to improve disease management and improve patients' quality of life.
4. A staff nurse as part of multi-disciplinary coronary care unit team has an important role in education patients and their families on the disease process. Management and control of symptoms and also providing support following diagnosis of cardiac disease.
5. Nurses are the integral providers involved in educating, coaching, monitoring and supporting patients and their families during the cardiac disease process. The staff nurse can assess the signs and symptoms of cardiac destabilization, provide emotional support, counseling, develop behavior modification techniques, monitor therapy compliance and also act as the healthcare

liaison for the patient and their family correctly after program.

6. The nurse as a patient educator' is one of the impediments to an effective teaching programme.
7. With regard to personal qualities of nurses after program, a significant evidence of improvement in personal characteristics of nurses (such as education, knowledge professional skills and training), in these two departments was found.
8. Further observation was found to be that any big gap between the training periods and practice can have some damaging consequences and it can affect their continuity of care, performance, motivation, decision making and most importantly their nursing concept during their practice.
9. Regular education, job training, meeting and seminars need to be provided as they are essential to keep their professional knowledge and performance up to date and at a high standard level.
10. Interval tests and training may be necessary for those nurses failing to meet the standard criteria in order to ensure a high quality of health care.

After program, nurses were skillful especially in early intervention when a patient shows signs of clinical instability, that is to reduce the incidence of complications and hence mortality.

In developing and transitional countries, however, coronary heart disease is increasing, partly as a result of increasing longevity, urbanization, and lifestyle changes. More than 60%

of the global burden of coronary heart disease occurs in developing countries. Must of the future increase in cardiovascular disease is expects to occur in developing countries (WHO, 2002).

2.9.1 Training and education

Most critical care nurses in the U.S. are registered nurses. Nurses in the US who wish to obtain cortical care nursing can do so through national advisory board, known as the American association of critical care nurses. This advisory board sets and maintains standards for critical care nurses. The certification offered by this board is known as critical care registered nurse (CCRN) as is popularly believed, but is merely certification as a critical care nurse for adult, pediatric, and neonatal population.

Registration is regularly term for the process that occurs between the individual nurses without specialty. However, the CCRN is an example of registration specialty certification in critical care.

Intensive care nurses are also required to be acquainted with wide variety of technology and its uses in critical care setting. This technology includes such equipments as hemodynamic and cardiac monitoring system, mechanical ventilator therapy, Intra-Aortic Balloon Pumps (IABP) Ventilatory Assist Devices (LVAD) and RVAD and continuous renal replacement equipment.

Usually the patients who are admitted to the I.C.U post-operative cardiac patient are post-coronary artery bypass craft, post valve replacement, or post congenital heart diseases repair.

This research focuses on the essential what, why, and who questions of post-operative cardiac patients assessment monitoring and therapeutic intervention.

The investigator chooses this research to provide nurses with information to enhance their critical care practice and so that they positively impact their patients from early detection or symptoms management to intervention that effects survival. American heart association (American heart association guidelines for cardiopulmonary resuscitation and emergency cardiovascular care-part 8, 2005).

Chapter Three Methodology

3.1 Study Design

Pre and post interventional prospective study that aimed to assess the effect of implementing training on the nurses' performance regarding open heart surgery.

3.2 Study Area

Khartoum state, Al Shaab and Ahmed Gasim cardiac centers.

Located in Khartoum state, it consists of different type of departments, an outpatient clinic, a laboratory, two theater rooms, a cath-lab, a coronary care unit, an intermediate care unit, a cardiac medical ward, a cardiac surgical ward, a neurosurgical ward and a neurosurgical ICU, an EEG department and an intensive cardiac care unit. The postoperative cardiac ICU in Al Shaab cardiac center is situated in close proximity to the sources of patient and services. And in a distinct area within the hospital, with controlled access, not through traffic to other departments supply and it is separated from the public traffic.

3.3 Study Population

The target population of the study were all intensive care nurses (98) who work in intensive care units in Al Shaab and Ahmed Gasim cardiac centers.

3.4 Inclusion Criteria

All nurses who are graduates and who work in an intensive care unit for more than 6 months.

3.5 Exclusion Criteria

Nurses who are employed in Al Shaab and Ahmed Gasim cardiac centers for a period of less than six months.

3.6 Sample Size

All nurses (a total of 98) who work in the intensive care units in Al Shaab and Ahmed Gasim cardiac centers, taken as the study group at the beginning of the study (phase 1) and assessed before intervention and the same group was assessed after intervention (phase 2) and then compared the results of the pre and post intervention.

3.7 Sampling Technique

Total converge sample.

3.8 Methods of Data Collection

A specifically designed questionnaire, an observation check list designed according to the standards that refer to American nurses association.

3.9 Operational Definitions of Demographic Variables

Every procedure should be done post operatively is a variable assess knowledge and performance regard to: patient endorsement, hemodynamic monitoring, treatment calculation and uses, care of invasive lines, arterial line, CVP line, arterial blood gases, measurement intake and output fluids and fluid replacement, care of underwater ceal, chest tube, care of ventilator, extubation, CPR (cardiac pulmonary resuscitation).

This operational definitions for variable used in main study.

Table (3.1): Operational Definitions of Variable

Variables	Operational definitions
1-Patient endorsement	Assessment and evaluation of patient when received to the ICU and write report about condition and dealing immediately with the patient According ABCS.
2-Hwmodynamic monitoring	Monitoring of vital organs post operatively, heart sound, respiratory rate, level of conscious
3-Treatment calculation	Calculate any drugs for support post operatively or with emergency Problem
4-Care of invasive lines	Care for intravenous line or central venous line or arterial

	line which support the patient post operatively
5-Measurement intake and output fluids	Measure any fluids intake through intravenous line or orally and fluid out the body should be measure to assess renal function.
6-Fluid replacement	Replacement of fluid loss according the volume of fluid loss through bleeding or vomiting.
7-Care of ventilator	Care of sealed drainage to avoid accumulation of fluid in the body and loading the heart.
8-Extubation	Care of the patient connected with artificial ventilating device as artificial lung to support oxygenation and exchange carbon dioxide. Mean switch from ventilator which done gradually after assessment.
9-Arterial blood gases	Patient fitness
10-CPR	Arterial blood sample taken to assess the fitness post operatively. Abbreviation of cardiopulmonary resuscitation Done for the patient when the heart stopping.

11-Oxygen administration	How the nurse administer oxygen for the patient (indication, devices, side effect)
12-Endotracheal suctioning	Tube inserted in trachea post-operative to maintain oxygenation through ventilator.

3.10 Study Instrument

Data collected using close ended, self-administrative interview guidance questionnaire which involve (45) question the answers evaluated by the score (poor for 25% correct answer, good for 50% correct answer and very good for 70% correct answers and excellent for more than 80% correct answers). The pre-test of questionnaire done in Al Shaab and Ahmed Gasim cardiac centers witch filling by investigator and well-trained monitors.

The evaluation of the practice done by observation check list to evaluate nurses performance with well-trained monitors.

3.11 Phases of The Study

1. Preparatory phase

Consent to conduct the study was taken from the responsible authorities of hospital after explanation of the aim of the study.

The learning program needs assessment sheet was development by the investigator based on the review of literature revised to the international training program for critical cardiac care nurses (American nurses association). Refer to cardiac surgeons in hospital and follow their observation on nurses practice and applied in learning program content. Verbal consent was obtained from nurses to participate in the study after explanation of the purpose of the study.

2. Educational program

Curriculum was developed by the investigator based on the recent standardized references in critical cardiac nursing (American nurses association) to promote nurses knowledge and practice. It included:

Three parts regaling knowledge (annexes 1).

-Part one
The aim and objective of training program:

- Introduction in anatomy and physiology of cardiovascular system.

- Part two

- Anatomy of respiratory system and respiratory problems (appendix).

- Part three
Procedure should be done in ICU post open-heart surgery (see appendix).

3.11.1 Phase 1 (Monitoring and Supervision Procedure)

A pilot study was carried out on 6 nurses who were working in cardiac word in Al Shaab & Ahmed Gasim cardiac centers before starting the actual data collection in order to identify the applicability and feasibility of tools in providing the requires data. Every nurse in ICU interviewed to assess their learning needs in regards to knowledge related to nursing management post open heart surgery.

Every nurse in study group was observed during routine application in ICU (intensive care unit) during every procedure to obtain data using specific design check list according to American Nurses Association Competency Test data was analyzed using the SPSS and the results of learning needs were identified by tool.

3.11.2 Phase 2 (Training)

Trainers were selected to share in training program after explanation of the study. The training team included professional expert in teaching and training.
- Cardiologist (Al Shaab teaching hospital).
- Cardiac surgeon (Al Shaab teaching hospital).
- Anesthetist (Al Shaab teaching hospital).
- Four especial ICU nurses two Sudanese one lecture in Rabat university the other responsible about nurses training in hospital.

Theoretical part was provided in the form of lectures. Seminars and video shows. It includes an important knowledge regarding intensive cardiac care unit. The practical part of training program was carried in the form of stations on different skills in continuous professional development center (CPDC)- the skill lab and intensive cardiac unit stations include activities regarding tool2 (procedures should be done post operatively, patient endorsement post operatively hemodynamic monitoring, care of central venous line. Care of arterial line, care of chest tube, endotracheal tube, intake and output fluid chart assessment, ABG sampling, care of patient during ventilator, weaning from ventilator, extubation from ventilator, equations of medications) the study group divided to four group and 4 stations every station take 45 minutes for three says. Skills in continuous professional development center (CPDC)-the skill lab and intensive cardiac care unit, regarding competency and case-based discussion. (Airway and oxygenation, breathing and ventilation, circulation, CPR, ECG, CXR, post open-heart surgery endorsement.

3.11.3 Phase 3 (Evaluation)

Nurses in study group were interviewed regarding cardiac surgery knowledge after intervention (training).

Monitors were dedicated to fill in the same observation check list that was used by the investigator in phase 1 (tool2) during morning and after the intervention (training).

Material and supplies were prepared sufficiently by the hospital authority throughout the period of data collection in both hospitals.

The study group was assessed three months after intervention to identify the impact of training on nurses using observation (check list).

Data was analyzed following the same process that was used in phase 1.

Data was categorized coded, summarized in master sheet then the result was presented in tables and graphs (computer).

3.12 Ethical Considerations

The research is respecting the rights of participants, treat data with confidentiality.

Verbal consents were obtained from all participants.

Letter was taken from university of all Gezira-faculty of medicine primary health center. Approval from administrative authorities of Al Shaab and Ahmed Gasim cardiac center was obtained.

3.13 Data Analysis

The data were analyzed by using statistical package for social sciences (SPSS) version 16 for quantitative data. Find out indicators aimed by this study such as knowledge. The difference in the performance between the study group before intervention and after intervention were assessed by mean of chi square significance was taken as $p<0.05$.

Statistical test. The study group was checked before and after implementation of the nursing intervention and then compare differences between both assessment data using significant test chi square.

Table (4.1) Effect of Training on Nurses Performance Regarding Gastrointestinal Procedures.

	Pre percent (%)				Post percent			
	Poor	Good	Very good	Excellent	Poor	Good	Very good	Excellent
NG tube insertion	28.6	57.1	14.3	0.0	0.0	0.0	71.4	28.6
a-tube feeding	0.0	0.0	28.6	71.4	0.0	0.0	28.6	71.4
c-paralyticileus	28.6	57.1	14.3	0.0	0.0	14.3	57.1	28.6
d-Gi bleeding	0.0	42.9	57.1	0.0	0.0	14.3	57.1	28.6
c-bowel obstruction	42.9	57.2	0.0	0.0	0.0	14.3	42.9	42.9

Mean less than 5
P value than 0.005

Table (4.2) Effect of Training on Nurses' Performance Regarding Urinary Procedures.

	Pre percent (%)				Post percent			
	Poor	Good	Very good	Excellent	Poor	Good	Very good	Excellent
Foley catheter insertion	0.0	28.6	42.9	28.6	0.0	28.5	71.5	0.0
Gu irrigation	0.0	42.9	28.6	28.6	0.0	42.9	57.1	0.0
Peritoneal dialysis	85.7	0.0	14.3	0.0	67.5	0.0	32.5	0.0
Hem dialysis	57.1	14.3	14.3	14.3	57.1	42.9	0.0	0.0
Electrolyte imbalance/replacement	0.0	0.0	71.4	28.6	0.0	84.5	14.5	0.0

Mean less than 5
P value than 0.005

Table (4.3) Effect of Training on Nurses' Performance Regarding Vascular Procedures.

	Pre percent (%)				Post percent			
	Poor	Good	Very good	Excellent	Poor	Good	Very good	Excellent
Peripheral pulses	28.6	57.1	14.3	0.0	0.0	0.0	14.3	28.6
Ultrasonic Doppler use	85.7	14.3	0.0	0.0	85.7	0.0	0.0	14.3
Start IV's	0.0	71.4	28.6	0.0	0.0	14.3	14.3	71.4
Central line maintenance	0.0	42.9	57.1	0.0	0.0	0.0	28.6	71.4
Infusion pumps	0.0	14.3	85.7	0.0	0.0	0.0	14.3	85.7
Administration of blood/blood product	0.0	42.9	57.1	0.0	0.0	0.0	42.9	57.1

Mean less than 5
P value than 0.005

Table (4.4) Effect of Training on Nurses' Performance Regarding Dressing Procedure.

	Pre percent (%)				Post percent			
	Poor	Good	Very good	Excellent	Poor	Good	Very good	Excellent
Change	0.0	100.0	0.0	0.0	0.0	0.0	0.0	100.0
Wound irrigation	0.0	57.2	42.8	0.0	0.0	0.0	14.3	85.7
Sterile dressing	0.0	85.5	14.5	0.0	0.0	0.0	0.0	100.0

Mean less than 5
P value than 0.00

Table (4.5) Effect of Training on Nurses' Performance Regarding Activities of Living.

	Pre percent (%)				Post percent			
	Poor	Good	Very good	Excellent	Poor	Good	Very good	Excellent
Safe environment	0.0	85.7	14.3	0.0	0.0	0.0	14.3	85.7
Communication and understanding	85.7	14.3	0.0	0.0	0.0	0.0	14.3	85.7
Eating and drinking	15.9	84.1	0.0	0.0	0.0	0.0	0.0	100.0
Personal hygiene	14.5	71.3	0.0	14.2	0.0	0.0	0.0	100.0
Mobilization	0.0	85.2	57.2	0.0	0.0	0.0	0.0	100.0
Physiotherapy	0.0	42.7	57.2	0.0	0.0	0.0	0.0	100.0
Daily sanitary	0.0	51.2	48.8	0.0	0.0	0.0	0.0	100.0
Reassurance	42.7	14.5	42.7	0.0	0.0	0.0	0.0	100.0
Condolences	85.5	14.5	0.0	0.0	0.0	0.0	28.6	71.4

Table (4.5) shows attitude of nurses regarding communication skills were poor at pre-intervention phase 85.7% while improved post-intervention 85% had an excellent score behavior. In same table regarding reassurance behavior of nurses with patient change to excellent behavior post intervention.

Chapter Four
Discussion

Open-heart surgery is a very serious surgery that needs professional and well-trained nursing staff in intensive cardiac unit.

This study was conducted to develop nurses expertise and in-depth understanding in the field of cardiovascular and thoracic nursing specifically in intensive cardiac care units. It will assist them to develop advance skills for nursing intervention in intensive care units.

The study was conducted over a three-year period (2010-2013). During this period, the investigator with the monitoring team observed the nurses performance during their shifts when they were handling their patients, through observation check list, on the other hand assessed their knowledge through special questionnaire designed according to the international nursing role regarding intensive cardiac nurse.

Since cardiac patients are very serious patients, nurse should be alert of them and should be able to process and analyze their patients' data to take timely proper decisions. This study aimed at assisting nurse to achieve this objective. First an intervention was conducted among 98 nurses (the total number of nurses in the two study cardiac centers: Al Shaab and Ahmed Gasim) to promote their knowledge and performance regarding open-heart surgery patients problem. Nursing role and timely decision making to avoid complications post-operatively.

The results, shown in figure (4.1), indicate that a large majority (86%) of nurses were disoriented about assessment of cardiac patients and did not do the procedures properly and in accordance with the ABCS endorsement of the patient post cardiac surgery. Nurses have to do many procedures post-operatively and have to assess patient airway, breathing and circulation, connect the patient with a ventilator to keep respiration and should write the operation history and the order for the patient if supported with medications or not, type of operation done for him or her, the investigations done and have to assess them immediately (Jaya, 2008). At pre intervention, the nurses' skills failed to follow faultless steps according to the international standard of nursing role in post open-heart surgery. But in post intervention, nurses training was highly significantly effective where 84% of them showed excellent skills $x2=196$, (p, value 0.000).

These findings are supported by Siley (2001) they stated that after program nurses were skillful especially in early intervention when a patient shows signs of clinical instability that is reduce the incidence of complication.

Mechanical ventilation is an artificial lung device connected to post-operative cardiac patients. Hemodynamic status, arterial blood gases should be assessed (Suzan,1995).

Figure (4.2) shown that most of nurses (69%) had good knowledge in pre intervention phase, it also explained that

(85%) of nurses improves their knowledge to very good scores in post intervention x2=196, (p, value 0.000).

Arterial blood gases is a sample taken from an arterial line closed sterile system connected to the monitor to observe arterial pressure on monitor and analyze regularly blood gases which assess oxygen saturation, carbon dioxide CO_2, HCO_3 ph electrolyte balance, any disturbances of this component will be fatal (Shila, 2001).

Figure (4.5) showed that a large percentage of nurses (67%) had a good knowledge regarding this procedure and upgrade, 85% had very good scores in post intervention while 2% had excellent cores. This means the training program is effective x2=196, (p value 0.000).

In same intervention training (Bartom, 2005) published in the American medical journal, maintain closed sterile drainage system at all time and proper hands washing before and after handling catheter tube & their tubing can prevent nosocomial infection.

Endotracheal is a tube intrachea to connect the patient with ventilator during the operation and post operation to maintain healthy tissue ventilation (Rokos & Bouthillet, 2007).

Figure (4.6) shows that slightly more than a half of the nurses (52%) had poor knowledge while a greater majority of nurses (86%) had an excellent score after post intervention while highlight, again it was an effective training program x2 196, (p, value 0.000).

Endotracheal tube and ventilator should be removed or extubate from cardiac surgery patient after 24 hours minimum post operatively to maintain respiratory system unless the patient is unfit, so the nurse should assess that patient and start weaning from ventilator through decreasing tidal volume or shift moods of ventilator gradually unit becoming sure the patient has fitness to extubate from ventilator (Rokos & Bouthillet, 2007).

Less than half of the nurses had poor skills regarding this procedure (40%) as shown in figure (4.9) while almost all of them (95%) improved to the level of very good skills, post intervention x2=196, (p, value 0.000).

Underwater sealed drainage is a tube inserted in mediastinum area post open cardiac surgery to remove residual blood or drainage, to prevent overload the chest cage and to maintain good function and good contraction of the heart to safe patient life (Caral, 2001).

Figure (4.10) showed statistically that exactly half of the nurse had poor performance regarding this procedure (50%). This percentage of nurses who improve performance in this procedure increased to (89%) in post intervention. That means effective training program. Under water sealed drain have to be removed when the drainage 0, after making sure that the patient has no complaints or complications after assessment of arterial blood gases and chest X-ray (Caral, 2001).

Figure (4.12) shows that more than half of nurses had a poor performance in pre intervention (56%) and only (42%) and only (42%) of them had good skills, but (67%) of them were ideally had a very good importance in post intervention x2=196, (p, value 0.000).

In same result about importance of training nurses and how the nursing intervention reduce UTI (urinary tract infection) if the nurse care to the folly catheter properly (Krumhols, 2009) had found a relationship between colonization and catheter related consequences including location.

Chest x-ray is procedure done for the patient immediately after operation to check operation and devices may be connected or inserted to support the heart. The nurse have to be alert regarding x-ray interpretation to take a timely discoing making to prevent any complications that may occur (pneomothorax, hemothorax or loss of lung volume) (Rokos & Bouthillet, 2007).

Figure (4.13) showed that more than half of nurses had good skills (61%) in pre intervention while the vast majority had an excellent score post intervention $x2=196$, (p, value 0.000).

Regarding cardiovascular system, the performance of nurses in arrhythmia as a complication post operatively which may lead to death, so the nurse have to be an expert to diagnose it immediately and timely, taking the decision to manage (Rokos & Bouthillet, 2007).

The majority of nurses (71.5%) had poor knowledge in the pre intervention phases, while in post intervention small change was achieved, as only 28% of the nurses had very good performance which means that they need more training regarding this problem, this topic is difficult and it need more time for reading but due to the time consuming in intensive cardiac care they were improves slightly.

Hemodynamc monitoring is a close observation of the patients which measures heart rate CVP, arterial blood pressure reparatory rate plus intake and output to maintain patient life and intervene immediately when the patient condition is not stable (Bartom, 2005).

More than half of nurses had poor performance in pre intervention as shown in figure (4.14) as the same time, the score improved vertically where more than half had an excellent attitude post intervention. X2=196, (p, value 0.000).

Some patients arrived to the intensive cardiac care unit from an open-heart surgery with supportive treatment for the heart to improve circulation for example adrenaline. The expert nurse knows how to assess the drug and how to be prepared to avoid complication (Giannuzzi et al., 2008).

In pre intervention phase (as shown in fig 14) more than half of nurses had either good or very good performance while in post intervention the percentage increased to 100% where all nurses had excellent performance x2=196, (p, value 0.000).

When a patient arrives to the intensive cardiac care unit and depends on ABC endorsement, the nurse should start with assessment of a lung sound systematically right and left side and be sure that the air is entering the lung, connect the monitor for patient with supported treatment if needed (Jaya, 2008). More than half of nurses (60%) had a very good performance regarding this activities, but after the intervention more than (80%) had very good performance as shown in figure (4.15).

According to the WHO, in 2002 7.2 million deaths worldwide resulted from coronary heart disease. In many developed countries, especially north American and western European countries coronary heart disease and resulting death rates are decreasing. This decrease is the result of improved prevention, diagnosis and treatment, particularly reductions in cigarette smoking, blood cholesterol and blood pressures. Importance of and B Harrison bellarmine college (Jaya, 2008).

Class glow coma scale is a procedure carried out to assess the consciousness level of patient, (Suzan,1995) this part of neurological of nurses on pre and post training program. At pre intervention more than half of nurses had a good performance whereas at post intervention the nurses performance goes further as 60% of them had a good very performance and 40% had an excellent performance which shows how an effective training program was x2=196 (p, value 0.000).

Dressing and solution is a very important part knowledge for nurses in order to look after cardiac patients. For protection from infection or septicemia which is fatal for cardiac patient. The nurse with mal practices can be a source of infection (Siley, 2001).

Table (4.4) shows that in pre intervention the majority of nurses had good performance which was absolutely due to the experience. The percentage was upgraded to 100% who were excellent in performance p value= 0.001.

Regarding communication skills nurses were poor at pre-intervention phase while improved post intervention 85% had an excellent score behavior promote to 100% post intervention had an excellent behavior post intervention show in table (4.5).

The success of this program was partially enhanced by the support of the managerial staff of the two hospitals.

Chapter Five
Conclusion and Recommendations

The study concluded that training as intervention was found the most influential factor regarding nurses' performance in open-heart surgery and technical nurses are able to provide an excellent service if trained, supervised well, and have incentives to practice properly.

6.1 Conclusion

The knowledge of most of nurses was improved after the training program especially with regards to definition, causes, risk factors, symptoms, and complications of disease.

Most of nurses in the hospital had more positive attitude regarding the effect of nursing knowledge in their performance.

The skills of nurses were improved after the training program especially with regards to devices (ventilator) of procedures (under water seal drain) regarding nursing management.

6.2 Recommendations

Based on the results of this study, the following recommendations are presented:

- Learning facilities such as library books and journals and the internet access regarding coronary artery disease, cardiac surgery patients care should be available for the nurses at hospital.
- Training program for all nurses working at the intensive cardiac unit on theoretical background, reasoning and operatively for every activity for each step in management of cardiac patient post aperatication for upgrading their knowledge and practices through more qualified nurses.
- Measures to introduce nursing management protocol in intensive cardiac care unit for nurses with continued in-service training.
- Proper and continuous supervision to assess the impact of training program on the nurses' performance.
- Standard log book for management of complication post open-heart surgery should be available in the intensive cardiac care unit.
- Periodic training program for critical cardiac nursing must be done as well as continuous monitoring and supervision for nurse's performance as a method of quality assurance.

Reference

American heart association guidelines for cardiopulmonary resuscitation and emergency cardiovascular care-part 8 (2005). Stabilization of the patient with acute coronary syndromes. Circulation 112: IV-89-IV-110.2005.

Bartom, M. M. (2005). Cardiovascular research journal. London. New York Elsevier B.V.

Caral T. (2001). Priscilla leane; "fundamental of nursing "United States of America; sixth edition; 2001; pp 66; pp 660-661.

Cabello J.B. burls A empstsnza J.I bayliss S. and Quinn T. (2010). "Oxygen therapy for acute myocardial infraction" Cochrane database syst rev 6.

Canto J.G Goldberg R.J hand M.M (2007) "Symptom presentation of women with acute coronary sysndromes: myth vs reality" arch. Intern. Med. 167 (22): 2405-13.

Gannuzzi, P, Temporellli, P. l and Marchioli R (2008). Global secondary prevention strategies to limit event recurrence after myocardial arch intern med. 2008 now 10;168 (20): 2194-204.

Jaya K.N (2008) "Essential of critical Care nursing"; first edition; New Delhi; medical publishers (p) LTD; pp: 122-123.

Krumholz, H (2009) "Patterns of hospital performance in acute myocardial infarction and heart failure- 30-day mortality and readmission". Circulation: cardiovascular quality and outcomes 2 (5): 407.

Lee, D, Kulick D. and Marks J (2006). Heart attack (myocardial infraction) by medicine net.com retrieved November 28,2006.

Rokos, I and Bouthillet T. (2007). "The emergency medical systems-to-balloon (E2B) challenge; building on the foundations of the D2B alliance" STEMI systems, issue two, may 2007, accessed June 16,2007.

Shila K.A. (2001). "Critical care nursing science & practices" second edition; London; 2001; pp:1-2. Pp:184-185.

Siley M. (2001). "Critical care secret"; second edition; pp:7-9.

Suzan, B.S. (1995). "Critical care reference"; third edition; London; st lovis philabelpia London; 1995;pp;480-482

WHO, (2002); integrated management of cardiovascular risk.

Appendices

University of Gazira
Primary health care and health education
Faculty of medicine
Study about promotion of nursing care in post open heart Surgery in Al Shaab and Ahmed Gasim cardiac centers Khartoum state (2012-2013)

Appendix (1)

Questionnaire

Can you kindly help me to answer my question completely?

Serial no:

Q1: Discuss immediate care post open heart surgery.

Q2: Discuss ways in which atelectasis can be minimize in the clinical setting.

Q3: Outline methods used to administer oxygen therapy.

Q4: Discuss humidification for a patient receiving supplemental oxygen.

Q5: Outline the difference between spontaneous breathing and positive pressure ventilation.

Q6: Identify the principles of mechanical ventilation.

Q7: Identify the indication of mechanical ventilation.

Q8: Discuss ventilation and perfusion relationships.

Q9: Identify the signs and possible causes of ventilator failure and its management

Q10: Describe modes and components of mechanical ventilation.

Q11: Describe the role of sedating analgesic and paralyzing agent in the management of a patient who mechanically ventilated.

Q13: outline the clinical effects of the following during groups that are relevant to their administration: narcotic, sedatives, hypnotics, local anesthetizes (LA).

Q14: Discuss complications of positive pressure ventilation.

Q15: Discuss complications of oxygen therapy.

Q16: How to asses a patient before and during the ventilation weaning process

Q17: Identify methods of weaning from positive pressure ventilation.

Q18: Describe indication of pulse oximetry.

Q19: Describe principles of pulse oximetry.

Q20: Describe waveforms of pulse oximetry.

Q21: Describe potential of inaccuracy of pulse oximetry.

Q22: Identify normal range values for the components of arterial blood gas.

Q23: Describe the various type of acid base disturbance in relation to arterial blood gases.

Q24: Identify the indications for endotracheal intubations.

Q25: Discuss the process for endotracheal intubations and the role of registers nurse.

Q26: Discuss the possible complication of endotracheal intubations and their collaborative management.

Q27: Discuss management of the patient who has an endotracheal tube.

Q28: Discuss management of the patient who has a tracheostomy tube.

Q29: Discuss the assessment criteria that would indicate a patient is ready for extubation.

Q30: Identify the patient presentation in failed extubation and discuss the collaborative management.

Q31: Discuss the indications for the use of underwater seal drains.

Q32: Discuss the principles and components of underwater seal drains.

Q33: Identify the potential complications associates with underwater seal drains.

Q34: Discuss the assessment and management of a patient with underwater seal drains.

Q35: Identify the assessment that would indicate underwater seal drains are ready to be removed.

Q36: Discuss a systematic process for interpretation of chest x-ray identifying tube/line placemen.

Q37: Discuss a systematic process for interpretation of chest x-ray identifying pneumothorax.

Q38: Discuss a systematic process for interpretation of chest x-ray identifying loss of lung volume.

ملحق (1.1): طريقة قياس الضغط الوريدي المركزي

- غسل الأيدي.
- شرح خطوات العمل للمريض.
- فتح جهاز الوريد المتصل بمحلول الملح ومسطرة القياس.
- تفريغ مسطرة القياس من الهواء عن طريق ملئها بمحلول الملح بواسطة فتح الحنفية الثلاثية بين محلول الملح والمسطرة، وغلقها على قسطرة الوريد المركزية.
- يتم التأكُّد من عمل قسطرة الوريد المركزية بكفاءة وذلك عن طريق سحب كمية صغيرة من الدم وحقنها في نفس الوقت.
- يتم غلق الحنفية الثلاثية على محلول الملح بعد التأكد من تفريغ الهواء كاملاً من المسطرة.

- يتم وضع المسطرة في نفس مستوى القلب عند منتصف خط الإبط.
- يتم فتح الحنفية الثلاثية بين المسطرة وقسطرة الوريد المركزية، ويلاحظ نزول السائل في المسطرة.
- يقرأ القياس عند ثباتِ السائل مع ملاحظة فصل المريض من جهاز التنفُّسِ الصناعي إذا كان متصلاً به، ويراعى أن يكون وضع المريض في السرير ثابتاً في كلِّ مرَّة ولم يتغير، ثم يتمُّ غلقُ الحنفية الثلاثية ناحية المريض لعدمِ السماح برجوع الدم من القسطرة.

طريقة قياس ضغط الدم الشرياني المباشر بواسطة جهاز المونيتور.

- غسل الايدي.
- شرح خطوات العمل للمريض.
- يتم فتح الحنفية الثلاثية المتصلة بالوصلة الشريانية وسحب 3 سم من الدم منها، ثم حقنها مرة أخرى.
- فتح جهاز الوريد المتصل بمحول الملح.

- فتح الحنفية بين الدوم وفتحة الحنفية على الهواء، ثم تسجيل الزيرو من على المونيتور، وعند ظهور الزيرو على المونيتور يتم غلق فتحة الحنفية على الهواء، وفتح الحنفية بين الوصلة الشريانية المتصلة بالمريض وفتحة الحنفية المتصلة بالدوم.
- يتم ظهور قياس ضغط الدم الشرياني المباشر بواسطة جهاز المونيتور.

الهدف:

التخلص من جميع السوائل والدم الموجود بالتجويف الصدري والحفاظ على قياس القلب والرئتين بوظائفهم بأعلى كفاءة ممكنة.

الأدوات المستخدمة:

- زجاجة محلول طبيعي 9% معقَّمة.
- وعاء مدرج خاص بتجميع الدم والسوائل.
- قفازات معقَّمة.
- شاش معقَّم وبلاستر.
- جِفت جراحي.
- بيتاين مطهر.

خطوات العمل:

- غسل الأيدي.
- شرح خطوات العمل للمريض.
- عمل الغيار اللازم مكان خروج الأنبوبة من صدر المريض بالبيتادين المطهِّر والشاش المعقَّم، ثم تغطيته بالبلاستر بعد التأكُّد مِن عَدَم وجود فتحات الأنبوبة والصدرية خارج جسم المريض.

- غلق الأنبوبة بواسطة الجفت الجراحي.
- فصل الوعاء الممتلئ وتفريغه من السوائل الموجودة فيه.
- غسل الوعاء بمحلول ملح معقِّم، ثم إضافة حوالي 200 سم من المحلول المعقِّم بحيث تكون فتحة نهاية الأنبوبة تحت مستوى سطح المحلول؛ وذلك لمنع دخول الهواء إلى التجويف الصدري.
- فتح الأنبوبة بواسطة الجفت الجراحي.
- التأكُّد من عمل الأنبوبة بكفاءة عن طريقة ملاحظة حركة السائل الموجود بها.
- عمل أشعة عادية على الصدر حسب أوامر الطبيب.

ملحق (2.1): العناية بمريض متَّصِل بقسطرة وريد مركزية

الهدف:

- قياس الضغط الوريدي المركزي.
- إعطاء الأدوية والمحاليل.

الأدوات المستخدمة:

- قسطرة وريد مركزي ذات مقياس مناسب (أحادية، ثنائية، أو ثلاثية الشعب).
- مسطرة قياس الضغط الوريدي المركزي.

- محلول ملح طبيعي 9% معقِّم، مضاف إليه أمبول هيبارين.
- قفازات معقَّمة، وحقنة أنسولين بها زيلوكين.
- شاش معقَّم وبلاستَر.
- بيتادين مطهِّر، وفوطة معقَّمة.
- حنفية ثلاثية على حسب عدد شعب قسطرة الوريد المركزية.
- مشرط جراحي معقَّم، وغرزة للتثبيت.
- حقنة 5 سم معقَّمة، وجهاز وريد معقَّم.

خطوات العمل:

- غسل الأيدي.
- شرح خطوات العمل للمريض.
- يتم ارتداء القفازات المعقمة، ثم فرش الفوطة المعقَّمة عند موضع تركيب قسطرة الوريد المركزية.

- تعقيم الجلد بالبيتادين عند موضع تركيب قسطرة الوريد المركزية.
- تركيب قسطرة الوريد المركزية بواسطة الطبيب بعد إعطاء الزيلوكين كتخدير موضعي، ثم تثبيتها بالغُرَز وتوصيل الحنفيات الثلاثية بشعب القسطرة، ثم وضع الشاش المعقم والبلاستر فوقَ مكان دخول القسطرة لتغطيته.
- يتم توصيل محلول ملح 9% معقم مضاف إليه أمبول هيبارين بجهاز الوريد، ويوصل بإحدى شعب القسطرة، ويتم توصيل مسطرة القياس بإحدى الفَتَحَات الأخرى للحنفية الثلاثية.

ملحق (3.1): العناية بالمريض على جهاز التنفس الصناعي

الهدَف:

استفادة المريض بأكبر قدرٍ ممكن من وجوده على جهاز التنفُّس الصناعي بأقلِّ المضاعفات المحتملة.

الأدوات المستخدمة:

1. زجاجة محلول ملح طبيعي 9%.
2. قسطرة شفط معقَّمة مقاسُها مناسب للأنبوبة الحنجرية.
3. حقنة 5 سم.

4. جهاز شفط بخراطيم شفط معقَّمة.
5. قفازات معقمة.
6. شاش معقَّم، بلاستر.
7. أمبوباج متَّصل بمصدر أكسجين.

خطوات العمل:

1. يتم تثبيت الأنبوبة الحنجرية جيداً مع معرفة الرقم المثبت عليها، وتدوينه في ملفِّ المريض.
2. يتم تغيير تثبيت الأنبوبة الحنجرية يومياً، أو حسب الحاجة لذلك.
3. ينظَّف الجلد جيداً حول الأنبوبة الحنجرية بالماء والصابون، ثم يجفَّف بشاشٍ مُعقَّم.
4. يتمُ غسلُ الأيدي، وارتداء القفازات المعقَّمة.
5. توصَلُ قسطرة الشَّفطِ بخرطومِ الشَّفط.
6. يفصل المريض عن الجِهاز، ويتمُّ الدخول بقسطرة وهي مغلقة بواسطة الضغط عليها بالأيدي، ويكون الدخول

بسرعة ورفق، ثمَّ تُرفَع الأيدي لتفتح القسطرة، ليتم الشفط، وتُسحب القسطرة ببطء وهي مفتوحة.

7. يتم غَسلُ قسطرة الشفط في محلول الملح المعقَّم.

8. يتم حقن 5 سم من محلول الملح في الأنبوبة الحنجرية، ثم يتمُّ التنفيخ بالأمبوباج؛ لإعطاء المريض أكسجين لمدة دقيقة أو أكثر حسب نسبة الأكسجين على المونيتور.

9. يكرَّرُ الشفط عِدَّة مرات، معَ ملاحَظَةِ لون الإفرازات وكمِّيتها ودرجة لزوجتها، مع تسجيل هذه الملاحظات في أوراق المريض.

10. يُغسَل الفم بماءٍ نظيف وقطعة شاش ملفوفة على خافض لسان، أو حقنة نظيفة.

ملحق (4.1): كيفية العناية بالجرح الناتج من إجراء عملية جراحية

الهدف:

منع تلوث الجرح بعد العملية.

الأدوات المستخدمة:

1. بيتادين مطهِّر، أو كحول طبِّي على حسب نوع الجرح.

1. جفنة معقَّمَة، وجفت معقَّم، وطينية معقمة.
2. شاش معقَّم وبلاستر وجوانتي معقَّم.

خطوات العمل:

1. غسل الأيدي.
2. شرح خطوات العمل للمريض مع الحفاظ على خصوصيته وكرامته.
3. التخلُّصُ من الغيار الموجود على الجرح.
4. وضع كمية من البتادين في الجفنة المعقَّمة.
5. وضعُ الشاش المعقَّم في الطينية المعقَّمة.
6. ارتداء القفازات.
7. الإمساك بالشاش المعقَّم بواسطة الجِفتِ المَعَقَّم.
8. غمرُ الشَّاشِ في البيتادين.
9. مسحُ الجُرحِ بالبيتادين من أعلى إلى أسفل في اتجاه واحد، دون العودة في الاتجاه المعاكس: (إذا كان الجرح طولياً) أو مسح الجرح بالبيتادين من الداخل إلى الخارج في اتجاه واحد مرة واحدة، دون العودة في الاتجاه المعاكس (إذا كان الجرح دائرياً) وتكرر هذه الخطوة أكثَرَ مِن مرة.
10. مسح الجلد بالبيتادين حول الجرح من أعلى إلى أسفل في اتجاه واحد مرة واحدة، دون العودة في الاتجاه المعاكس

(إذا كان الجرح طولياً).. نبدأ بالناحية الأبعد أولاً، ثم الأقرب بعد ذلك.

11. مسح الجلد بالبيتادين حول الجرح من الخارج في اتجاه واحد مرة واحدة دون العودة في الاتجاه المعاكس (اذا كان الجرح دائريا).

12. مسح البيتادين من على الجرح بواسطة الشاش المعقَّم من أعلى إلى أسفل في اتجاه واحد مرة واحدة دون العودة في الاتجاه المعاكس (اذا كان الجرح طوليا) أو مسح البيتادين من الداخل الى الخارج في اتجاه واحد مرة واحدة دون العودة في الاتجاه المعاكس (إذا كان الجرح دائرياً).

13. مسح الجلد بالشاش المعقَّم حول الجرح من أعلى إلى أسفل في اتجاه واحد، دون العودة في الاتجاه المعاكس (إذا كان الجرح طولياً) نبدأ بالناحية الأبعد أولاً، ثم الاقرب بعد ذلك.

14. مسح الجلد بالشاش المعقَّم حول الجرح مِن الخارج في اتجاه واحد مرة واحدة، دون العودة في الاتجاه المعاكِس (إذا كان الجرح دائرياً).

15. تغطية الجرح بالشاش المعقَّم والبلاستر.
16. يجب ملاحظة الجرح دائما من حيث حدوث نزيف أو تغير لون الجلد حول الجرح.

ملحق (5.1): طريقة قياس الضغط الوريدى المركزي

17. غسل الأيدي.
18. شرح خطوات العمل للمريض.
19. فتح جهاز الوريد المتصل بمحلول الملح ومسطرة القياس.
20. تفريغ مسطرة القياس من الهواء عن طريق ملئها بمحلول الملح بواسطة فتح الحنفية الثلاثية بين محلول الملح والمسطرة وغلقها على قسطرة الوريد المركزية.
21. يتم التأكد من عمل قسطرة الوريد المركزية بكفاءة وذلك عن طريق سحب كمية من الدم وحقنها في نفس الوقت.
22. يتم غلق الحنفية الثلاثية على محلول الملح بعد التأكُّد من تفريغ الهواء كاملاً من المسطرة.

23. يتم وضع المسطرة في نفس مستوى القلب عند منتصف خط الإبط.

24. يتمُّ فتحُ الحنفية الثلاثية بين المسطرة وقسطرة الوريد المركزية، ويلاحظ نزول السائل في المسطرة.

25. يُقرَأ القياس عند ثبات السائل مع ملاحظة فصل المريض مِن جهاز التنفس الصناعي، إذا كان متصلاً به، ويراعى أن يكون وضع المريض في السرير ثابتاً في كل مرة ولم يتغيَّر، ثم يتمُّ غلقُ الحنفيَّة الثُّلاثيَّة مِن ناحية المريض لعدم السَّماح برجوع الدم من القسطرة.

ملحق (6.1): العناية بمريض متصل بقسطرة وريد مركزية

الهدف:

قياس الضغط الوريدي المركزي.

إعطاء الأدوية والمحاليل.

الأدوات المستخدمة:

1. قسطرة وريد مركزي ذات مقياس مناسب (أحادية، ثنائية، أو ثلاثية الشعب).
2. مسطرة قياس الضغط الوريدي المركزي.
3. محلول ملح طبيعي 9%، معقَّم، مُضافٌ إليه أمبول هيبارين.

4. قفازات معقَّمة وحقنة أنسولين بها زيلوكين.
5. شاش معقَّم وبلاستَر.
6. بيتادين مطهِّر وفوطَة معقَّمَة.
7. حنفية ثلاثية على حسب عددِ شُعَب قسطرة الوريد المركزية.
8. مشرط جراحي مُعَقَّم، وغرزة للتثبيت.
9. حقنة 5سم معقَّمة، وجهاز وريد مُعقَّم.

خطوات العمل:

1. غسل الأيدي.
2. شرح خطوات العمل للمريض.
3. يتم ارتداء القفازات المعقَّمة، ثم فرش الفوطة المعقَّمة عند موضع تركيب قسطرة الوريد المركزية.
4. تعقيم الجلد بالبيتادين عند موضع تركيب قسطرة الوريد المركزية.
5. تركيب قسطرة الوريد المركزية بواسطة الطبيب بعد إعطاء الزيلوكين كتخديرٍ موضعي، ثم تثبيتها بالغُرَز،

وتوصيل الحنفيات الثلاثية بشُعَب القسطَرة، ثمَّ وضعُ الشاش المعقَّم والبلاستر فوق مكان دخول القسطرة لتغطيته.

6. يتم توصيل محلول ملح 9%، معقم، مضاف إليه أمبول هيبارين بجهاز الوريد، ويوصل بإحدى شُعَب القسطرة، ويتم توصيل مسطرةِ القياس بإحدى الفتحات الأخرى للحنفية الثلاثية.

ملحق (7.1): العناية بمريض متصل بكانيولا شريانية

الهدف:

1. قياس ضغط الدم الشرياني المباشر.
2. سحب عينات غازات الدم.

الأدوات المستخدمة:

1. كانيولا ذات مقياس مناسب للمريض.
2. قفازات معقمة.
3. قطن مضاف إليه كحول طبي وبلاستر للتثبيت.
4. حنفية ثلاثية، ووصلة شريانية.

5. حقنة 5سم وجهاز وريد.
6. دوم وترانسديوسر مناسبة لجهاز المونيتور.

خطوات العمل:

1. غسل الايدي.
2. شرح خطوات العمل للمريض.
3. يتم ارتداء القفازات المعقَّمة، ثم تعقيم الجلد بالقطن المضاف إليه كحول عند موضِع تركيبِ الكانيولا.
4. يتم إدخالُ الكانيولا في الشريان، ثم يتمُّ توصيلها بالوصلة الشريانية، ويتمُّ اختبار عملها بكفاءة عن طريق ملاحظة رجوع الدم في الوصلة الشريانية.
5. يتم توصيل إحدى الحنفيات الثلاثية بالوصلة الشريانية وجهاز الوريد المتصل بزجاجة محلول الملح، والحنفية الأخرى توصل بالدم.
6. تثبيت الكانيولا بواسطة البلاستر، ويكتب عليه تاريخ التركيب، ثم يتم تغيير البلاستر يومياً، مع تنظيف الجلد

حول موضِع دخول الكانيولا بواسطة الدَّخلِ المضاف إليه كحول.

7. يجب ملاحظة وجود أيّ تورُّم أو تغيُّر لونِ الجلد عند موضع دخول الكانيولا، ففي هذه الحالة يجب إبلاغ الطبيب وخلعها حالاً.

8. يجب الحفاظ على مكان وجود الكانيولا نظيفاً وجافاً دائماً.

9. يجب الحفاظ على غلق الحنفية الثلاثية باستمرار؛ وذلك في حالة عدم استخدامها، مع مسح فتحاتها بكحول عند استخدامها.

ملحق (8.1): طريقة قياس ضغط الدم الشرياني المباشر بواسطة جهاز المونيتور

1. غسل الأيدي.
2. شرح خطوات العمل للمريض.
3. يتم فتح الحنفية الثلاثية المتَّصِلة بالوصلة الشريانية وسحب 3سم من الدم منها، ثم حقنها مرة أخرى.
4. فتح جهاز الوريد المتَّصِل بمحلول الملح.
5. فتح الحنفية بين الدوم وفتحة الحنفية على الهواء، ثم تسجيل الزيرو مِن على المونيتور، وعند ظهور الزيرو على المونيتور يتمُّ غلق فتحة الحنفية على الهواء، وفتح الحنفية بين الوصلة الشريانية المتَّصِلة بالمريض وفتحة الحنفية المتصلة بالدوم.

6. يتم ظهور قياس ضغط الدم الشرياني المباشر بواسطة جهاز المونيتور.

ملحق (9.1): العناية بمريض متصل بأنبوبة صدرية

الهدف:

التخلُّص من جميع السوائل والدم الموجود بالتجويف الصدري، والحفاظ على قيامِ القلبِ والرئتين بوظائفهم بأعلى كفاءة ممكنة.

الأدوات المستخدمة:

1. زجاجة محلول طبيعي 9% معقمة.
2. وعاء مدرج خاص بتجميع الدم والسوائل.
3. قفازات معقَّمة.
4. شاش معقم وبلاستر.

5. جِفت جراحي.
6. بيتايِن مطهِّر.

خطوات العمل:

1. غسل الأيدي.
2. شرح خطوات العمل للمريض.
3. عمل الغيار اللازم مكان خروج الأنبوبة من صدرِ المريض بالبيتادين المطهِّر والشاش المعقَّم، ثم تغطيته بالبلاستر بعدَ التأكُّد مِن عدمِ وجود فتحتي الأنبوبة والصدرية خارج جسم المريض.
4. غلق الأنبوبة بواسطة الجِفت الجراحي.
5. فصل الوعاء الممتلئ وتفريغه من السوائل الموجودة به.
6. غسلُ الوعاء بمحلول ملح معقَّم، ثم إضافة حوالي 200 سم مِن المحلول المعقَّم بحيثِ تكون فتحة نهاية الأنبوبة تحت مستوى سطح المحلول وذلك لمنع دخول الهواء الى التجويف الصدري.

7. فتح الأنبوبة بواسطة الجفت الجراحي.
8. التأكد مِن عمَل الأنبوبة بكفاءة عن طريق ملاحظة حركة السائل الموجود فيها.
9. عمل أشعة عادية على الصدر حسب أوامر الطبيب.

Appendix (2)
Observation Checklist

Nursing performance regarding Cardiovascular system

	Pre intervention			
	Poor	Good	Very good	Excellent
Arrhythmia analysis				
Lead ECG interpretation-12				
Defibrillation/cardiovertion				
Hemodynamic monitoring				
Arterial line (transducer set up)				
SPO2 monitoring				
Assist with central line insertion				

e-pre/post cardiac surgery endorsement				
f-ventricular assist device				
A-atropine				
b-thrombolytic				
c-adrenaline				

Nursing skills regarding respiratory nursing procedures (pre)

	Percent (%)			
	Poor	Good	Very good	Excellent
Assessment lung sound				
Establish airway				
Assist with intubation				
Assist with extubation				
Pulse oximetry				
Incentive spirometry				
02 administration				

Obtain ABG results				
a-chest tube removal				
b-trachestomy removal				
h-pre/post thoracic surgery assessment				
i-ventilator (A/C, IMV, PEEP)				
j-weaning parameters (pressure support, (CPAP)				
a-aminopyline				
b-corticosteroids				
e-nebulizer treatment				

Nursing skills regarding neurological system

	Percent (%)			
	Poor	Good	Very good	Excellent
Perform neuron assessment				
Glasgow coma scale				

Assist with lumbar puncture				
Care of patient with seizure activity and precaution				
a-dexamethasone				
b-phyntoin				
c-magnesium sulfate				
d-midazolam				
e-ephenobarbital				
f-steroids				
g-diazepam				

Nursing skills regarding Gastrointestinal system

	Percent (%)			
	Poor	Good	Very good	Excellent
NG tube insertion				
a-tube feeding				
c paralyticileus				
d-Gi bleeding				
e-bowel obstruction				

Nursing skills regarding Genitourinary system

	Percent (%)			
	Poor	Good	Very good	Excellent
Poley catheter				
Gu irrigation				
Peritoneal dialysis				
hemodialysis				
Electrolyte imbalance/replacement				

Nursing skills regarding vascular system

	Percent (%)			
	Poor	Good	Very good	Excellent
Peripheral pulses				
Peripheral pulses				
Start IV's				
Central line maintenance				
Infusion pumps				
Administration of blood/blood produce				

Nursing skills regarding Dressing/drains

	Percent (%)			
	Poor	Good	Very good	Excellent
Change				
Wound irrigation				
Sterile dressing				

Nursing skills regarding Activities of living

	Percent (%)			
	Poor	Good	Very good	Excellent
Safe environment				
Communication and understanding				
Eating and drinking				
Personal Hygiene				
Mobilization				
Physiotherapy				
Daily sanitary				
Reassurance				
Condolences				

ملحق (1.2): قائمة مراجعة لتقييم أداء الممرضات في العلامات الحيوية

نقاط التقييم	اليوم الأول		اليوم الثاني		اليوم الثالث		اليوم الرابع		اليوم الخامس		اليوم السادس	
	نعم	لا	نعم	لا	نعم	لا	نعم	لا	نعم	لا	نعم	لا
1. هل قامت الممرضة بشرح الإجراء التمريضي للمريض/ة قبل القيام به؟												

4.هل قامت الممرضة بغسل	3.هل راعت الممرضة خصوصية وكرامة المريض/ة	2.هل قامت الممرضة بتحضير كل ما تحتاجه لإجراء المطلوب القيام به؟

المرض/قبل وبعد التعامل مع بدءا (روتيني) قبل						

ملحق (2.2): التنفس وقياس ضغط الدم

نقاط التقييم	اليوم الأول		اليوم الثاني		اليوم الثالث		اليوم الرابع		اليوم الخامس		اليوم السادس	
	نعم	لا	نعم	لا	نعم	لا	نعم	لا	نعم	لا	نعم	لا
التنفس												
1. هل تم قياس التنفس خلال ستين ثانية؟												
2. هل سرعة التنفس تم تدوينها بطريقة صحيحة بورقة المشاهدات؟												

7.هل تم استعمال القياس الصحيح لل(Cuff)؟	5.هل قامت الممرضة بوضع المرضى/العميل في الوضع المطلوب؟	5.هل قامت الممرضة بوضع المرضى/العميل في الوضع المطلوب؟	4.هل قامت الممرضة بفحص الجهاز قبل استعماله؟	قياس ضغط الدم	3.هل تم تقييم نوع سرعة عمق وطريقة التنفس؟

8. هل تم قياس ضغط الدم سابقاً.. هل أحسَت المريضة النبض؟	9.هل تم نفخ ال (cuff) من 20 إل 30 ملم زئبقي فوق آخر قراءة؟	10.هل تم تدوين القراءة ومقارنتها بالقياسات السابقة؟	11.هل تم تنظيف الجهاز بعد الاستعمال

ملحق (2.3): قائمة مراجعة لتقييم أداء الممرضات في الإنقاذ عن طريق إنعاش القلب (فردان)

نقاط التقييم	اليوم الأول		اليوم الثاني		اليوم الثالث		اليوم الرابع		اليوم الخامس		اليوم السادس		الأسباب
	نعم	لا	نعم	لا	نعم	لا	نعم	لا	نعم	لا	نعم	لا	
وصول المنقذ الثاني بجهاز الصدمات الكهربائية مع عدم توقف المنقذ الأول بعملية إنعاش القلب													
1. هل قام المنقذ بتشغيل جهاز الصدمات الكهربائية؟													

3. هل قام المنفذ بإخلاء المرضى من الحيطان والمصدر (الشاك) لعمل صدمة كهربائية؟	2. هل قام المنفذ باختيار البادات المناسبة ووضعها في أماكنها الصحيحة؟

5. هل قام المنقذ الثاني بعمل الضغط بالمعدل الصحيح؟	4. هل قام المنقذ الثاني باستكمال إنعاش القلب بعد الصدمة الكهربائية الأولى؟

المنقذ الثاني يستكمل إنعاش القلب والمنقذ الأول يستكمل عملية التنفس الصناعي

Appendix (3)
Education Program

Course name: intensive care and emergency life support course for nurses

Course duration :3days

Course equipments:

- CPR manikins.
- Always adjuncts.
- ALS manikins + simulators.

Clinical materials:

- Course manual.
- Lectures (power point).
- Scenarios.

Competency statements (objectives):

*Airway and oxygenation

The trainee:

- Describes the signs of airway obstruction.
- Demonstrates safe use of simple airway maneuvers/ adjuncts (head-tilt, chin lift, suction, oropharyngeal, nasopharyngeal airway)
- Describe the indications and rationale for safe oxygen therapy in the critically ill patient.
- Demonstrates basic treatment for simulated choking.

*Breathing and ventilation

The trainee:

- Demonstrates a systematic clinical assessment of breathing and oxygenation.
- Describe the common causes of breathlessness.
- Describe the clinical signs and treatment of a tension pneumothorax.
- Demonstrates effective bag-mask ventilation.
- Demonstrates effective mouth-mask ventilation.
- Demonstrates effective expired air ventilation without adjuncts.

*Circulation

The trainee:

- Describe the clinical features of shock.
- Describe potentially reversible causes of a cardiac arrest.
- Demonstrates the immediate management of a simulated witnesses in-hospital cardiac arrest.
- Describe how to recognize and treat common peri-arrest arrhymias.
- Demonstrates peripheral venous annulations including attention to patient comfort and infection control.
- Demonstrates effective external chest compression.
- Describes effective fluid resuscitation.
- Describes control of external hemorrhage.
- Recognize cardiac arrest rhythms (VF, pulseless VT, PEA, and asystole).
- Demonstrates safe and effective use of an automated external defibrillator.
- Demonstrates safe and effective use of a manual defibrillator.

*Confusion and coma

The trainee

- Describes the common causes of altered consciousness.
- Demonstrates a systematic approach to the assessment of the acutely ill patient with altered consciousness.

- Describes how to recognize and initiate treatment of status epilepticus.
- Demonstrates the recovery position.

*Drugs therapeutics and protocols

The trainee

- Describes how to recognize and initiate treatment for an acute of asthma.
- Describes how to recognize and initiate treatment for diabetic emergencies.
- Describes how to recognize and initiate treatment for acute heart failure.
- Describes how to recognize and initiate treatment for and anaphylactic reaction.
- Describes the causes, presentation and treatment of oliguria.
- Describes the indications and dosages of drugs used in the management of a cardiac arrest.
- Describes how to recognize and initiate treatment for septicemia & septic shock.
- Describes how to recognize and initiate treatment for common drug overdoses.
- Describes how to recognize and initiate treatment for acute coronary syndromes.
- Describes the role of vasoactive drugs in treatment of the shocked patient.

*Clinical examination, monitoring and investigations

The trainee

- Describe normal physiological anges for basic vital signs including pulse, blood, pressure, SpO2, respiratory rate, urine output and body temperature.
- Demonstrates a systematic approach to the clinical assessment and timely management of the critically ill patient.
- Describe the importance of repeated and timely reassessment of the acutely ill patient.
- Describe appropriate laboratory tests for the initial investigation of the acutely ill patient.

*Team working, organization and communication

The trainee

- Describe/ Demonstrates how to recognize one's own limitations and when to call for help.
- Describe/ Demonstrates the principles of good communication skills.
- Demonstrates the ability to work as part of a multi-professional team.
- Demonstrates the role of early warning sconing systems and/or CU outreach.
- Demonstrates good time keeping, punctuality.

*Patient and societal needs

The trainee

- Describes the importance of and methods for achieving adequate pain control.

*Trauma

- Describes the principles of recognition and initial management of patients with suspected head injuries.
- Describes of demonstrates a systematic approach to assessment and immediate treatment of the victim of trauma.

*Equipment

- Demonstrates how to set up and give high flow and controlled oxygen therapy correctly.

*Infection and inflammation

The trainee

- Describes the recognition and immediate resuscitation of a patient with sepsis.
- Describes a rational approach to antibiotic prescribing in the patient with sepsis.

*Course components

- Lectures.
- Skill station.
- Clinical scenarios.
- Pre-course assessment (MCQs)-3 week before the course.
- Continuous assessment (skill &commitments).
- Post-course assessment (MCQs).
  New instructor pathway

1-Pass the whole assessment part (IP).
2-Attend & pass clinical instructor course (IC).
3-Attend at least 2 courses with continuous evaluation from the senior instructors.
4-Final approval from the course director.

Note

The course is designed to develop the fundamental competencies and skills required to save, stabilize initially mange the acutely and critically ill patients, it almost covered whole the ICU and ER cases.

Basic assessment & support seriously ill patient in developing health care systems

This course is designed to teach acute medicine to doctors practicing in health care systems with limited resource

Topic includes:
      1-Assessment of the seriously ill patient
      2-Always management & always obstruction

3-Acute respiratory failure
4-ECG interpretation.
5-Life threatening arrhythmias.
6-Shock
7-Fluid replacement
8-Metabolic and electrolyte disturbances
9-Oliguria and acute renal failure
10-Neurological emergencies
11-Server trauma
12-Infection control
13-Sepsis
14-Choosing antibiotics

Skill stations and cases-based discussion

1-Always management
2-CPR and safe defibrillation
3-ECG interpretation
4-ABG interpretation
5-CXR interpretation
6-Sepsis cases discussion
7-Post open heart surgery endorsement

Cont. Appendix (3.1)
Continuing Professional Development Center

Schedule of Training Program

Day (1)

time	topic	Instructor

Day (3)

time	topic	Instructor
Lectures		
8:30-9:00	Disability injuries	Course instructor
Clinical scenarios		
9:00-9:20	Head injuries	Course instructor
9:20-9:40	Seizures	Course instructor
9:40-10:00	Acute confessional staus	Course instructor
10:00-10:20	Hypo & hyperglycemia	Course instructor
10:20-10:40	Oliguria	Course instructor
10:40-11:10	Breakfast	
11:10-11:40	Team work & communication	Course instructor
Clinical scenarios		
11:40-12:00	Drugs overdose	Course instructor
12:00-12:20	Recognition of your own limits	Course instructor
12:20-12:45	Feedback & closure	Course instructor
12:45-13:25	Exam	Course instructor
13:25	End of the course	Course instructor